No More Excuses!

Choose to be fit, healthy, and happy

TAWNI GOMES

PAPER
CHASE
PRESS

New Orleans, LA

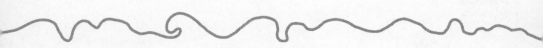

This book is dedicated to Oprah and Grandma Lois
for showing me a better way to live my life

mind body spirit

ACKNOWLEDGEMENTS

I've been writing my acknowledgements for this book before I ever started writing the first chapter. I am a firm believer in surrounding yourself with people that believe in you. I have the BEST Cheerleaders in the world!

These are in no particular order of importance, but I want to thank:

Oprah Winfrey and Bob Greene for writing the book *Make the Connection* and being my inspiration to finally GET RID OF MY EXCUSES once and for all. It's been a real privilege to carry your message. You have saved my life more than once. I will be eternally grateful. You are a national treasure! I could write an entire book of how grateful I am to you and all the lessons I've learned and continue to learn from you. You make me want to be a better person.

My husband, Martin for believing in me and telling me if I was going to quit my job to write the book, I'd have to learn to live without my daily stop at Starbucks. And for making the necessary financial sacrifices for me to quit my job to write this book. You are a quiet giant! Thank you for showing me what love is all about.

Amby Burfoot, editor of *Runner's World* Magazine for publishing the article on the Connectors in the February 1999 issue. It was THAT single issue that transformed the Connectors to the international group they are today. That was business. But, on a personal side you have always answered my emails and phone calls and ALWAYS made me feel important and special.

My very patient editor Jennifer. This book wouldn't make sense without your strong sense of order. I am grateful for your never ending cheerleading and support for me and this project.

Werner, my publisher for being so flexible with me as a first time author.

Jeff Galloway for leading the way for the beginners in the world. You are so generous in spirit and I'm grateful for the knowledge and friendship you have shared with me.

John "the penguin" Bingham for always making me laugh when all I want to do is cry. I am amazed I can run for 2 hours with you and feel refreshed and ready to do it all over again. I appreciate your support and always look forward to our chats.

Scott Hublou, founder of Asimba.com for allowing the CONNECTORS to have a great way to train for all of their events. And for being a great ear for me to bend in those rough beginning months. Thank you for being a great example of taking care of the BIG ROCKS in life.

T.P., for being a great friend and putting up with all my late night phone calls! Your assistance with the technical support for the website has been a GODSEND! You are an angel. I couldn't have created this network without you. (that's an UNDERSTATEMENT!)

The "Brians" in my life. Each of you hold a special place in my heart. Thank you for believing in me no matter what.

My A.D. what a gift you are in my life!

Lyle for teaching me some very valuable lessons.

Cynthia Kersey, author of *Unstoppable* for listening to me and believing in me.

My good friends Debbie, Ellen, Nan, Martha, Barb, Karen and Chris: Ladies, you are truly my INSPIRATION. Your example of determination and courage has gotten me out of bed more than once! Thank you for your tremendous friendships.

Megan for your incredible writing style and countless interviews and phone calls to get my story told more than once.

All of my Connector Leaders throughout the world who without any money lead the local groups everyday and keep me informed of the latest happenings with the local Connector groups.

And of course all the CONNECTORS out there who are literally the wind beneath my wings and the MAIN reason I agreed to do this book. I can't wait to meet all of you in person soon. I appreciate all of you encouraging me every step of the way along this journey. Everyday I am inspired by each of you.

mind body spirit

Contents

mind body spirit

It takes courage to change your life. Until I was in my early 30s, I didn't think I had enough courage to make any significant changes in the way I lived. But in 1996, when I looked honestly at myself for the first time, accepted the fact that I was carrying almost 300 pounds on a 5'5" frame, and realized that I was the only person in the world who could do anything about it, I found courage that I never knew I had.

Maybe you feel that you don't have enough courage either. Maybe, like I did for so many years, you look for excuses to explain your weight and the reasons why you don't walk to the post office, don't buy healthy food at the grocery store, and don't drive by the ice cream shop without stopping. But I've come to realize that excuses are just a mask, a little psychological trick that we use to hide from ourselves and to turn over responsibility to other people or to external events. To change your life, you have to be the one in control, and that means being totally honest with yourself and throwing all those maybes, all those excuses, and all that blame out the window. Believe me, the courage is inside you—even if you don't feel very brave right now. Remember that old saying, "The longest journey begins with a single step"? If you look at your journey as a single step and not as an overwhelming challenge, that first step doesn't seem very hard. And then the second step just naturally follows the first. The process keeps going bit by bit until one day you realize just how far you've come.

Today's the day you can take that first step. And you don't have to do it alone. A nationwide network of supportive people—all on the same journey—is waiting for you and ready to help in any way they can. These wonderful people are the Connectors, thousands of men and women across the

mind body spirit

country who have made the decision to change their lives and who gather at my web site, connectingconnectors.com, to share their struggles, to encourage each other, and to celebrate their successes. This kind of support is invaluable, providing a sounding board for those times when you doubt your conviction and offering an enthusiastic cheering section when you meet one of your goals.

I wish I had such a group when I began my journey. I started alone when I decided that September day in 1996 to take charge of my life. Little by little, I began to change the way I ate and I started exercising—tentatively at first with brief stretches on the treadmill and then with longer walks outside. Just three months after I began my new lifestyle, I was struck and badly injured by a car while I was on one of my daily walks. Sticking with my program after the accident was a real challenge. Not only did I have to find new ways to exercise, but I also had to overcome the biggest temptation of all—making excuses for not exercising. I knew I needed help to keep going and I turned to the Internet, eventually developing a group of women around the country who also wanted to make permanent changes in their lives to live life fit and happy. With the support of these women, I recovered from my accident, continued my eating and exercise program, and step-by-step, I began to run—literally. I started my journey with labored, halting steps and I am now a marathon runner, more than 100 pounds lighter, and more fit and happy than I have ever been in my life.

That small group of supportive women who helped me so much has grown into the Connectors, more than 20,000 strong, who receive my "Thought for the day" messages and are an ongoing source of inspiration for everyone who joins us on our journey. I feel like we Connectors are all one big family because our interaction is not limited to cyberspace. Designated regional contacts help organize local Connectors activities and events. Whenever I travel to a marathon or other event, I always make sure to get together with Connectors in the area.

I want everyone to know about the Connectors and the wonderful support they provide. I've shared my enthusiasm about the Connectors on radio talk show programs, in newspaper and magazine interviews, on Web sites, and even on *Oprah*. And that's why I've written this book—to let you know about these marvelous people and how much they can help you find the courage you have within you.

Throughout this book I have included many inspiring stories from the Connectors. And to a large extent, this book is as much their story as it is my own. We want to share with you the successes we have all had together as we make significant changes in our lives. We want you to understand that every step counts no matter how big or small. In these pages, we share our personal challenges and setbacks. We tell you the baby steps we have taken and how we stayed motivated. We tell you what worked for us and what did not. We discuss the right attitude and frame of mind you need, what types of exercises you may want to consider, the best foods to eat, and how you can get support.

You can believe in yourself, and you can do it. You have what it takes right now to change your life, and we are there every day to help you see it through. If changing your life means losing weight and getting fit, you can do that. If changing your life means developing the self-confidence to do things for your family and for your community, you can do that too. You can do whatever you want, no matter what your past experience has been. Sooner or later, we all face a new day when we realize that the future can be anything we want it to be.

It's my hope that this book will help you reach the same point that the Connectors and I have all reached, or are in the process of reaching: we control our own lives and will accept no more excuses! This is the place where real change begins to happen—not just in your life but in the lives of others as well. I truly believe we make this world just a little better if each of us works on ourselves. Because if you work to improve yourself, you are in a better position to help others. And that is what I believe life is about. I wish you the very best life and successes!

Love,

Tawni

mind   body   spirit

Long way from home

All my life I've wanted to matter. Really matter. Maybe all my pain and suffering will serve a greater good. Just thinking that this will all matter at a later time gets me through this ordeal.

JOURNAL ENTRY, JANUARY 12, 1997

They tell me I was hit by a car. They say I flew about 50 yards through the early morning air in San Francisco, the sun just breaking on a new day. They say the driver never saw me. I believe them, but I don't have any memory of it. Although my body reminds me it happened when I am sore or take longer to heal after running, no nightmares that wake me up in the middle of the night, the fading echoes of a roaring engine in my ears.

I woke up in the emergency room at Seton Hospital. Naked and lying on a hard board to keep my back straight, I watched as a team of emergency people brought in someone who had been beaten with a baseball bat. She was obviously the priority here. Nevertheless, I panicked and screamed to the nurse that the back of my head was bleeding, that blood was pouring down my back. It was sweat.

They cut off my clothes and examined me. "Does this hurt? How about this?" I pulled up the sheets after they had retreated, deciding I wasn't a life or death case. Looking down at my toes, I tried to make them wiggle. If my toes could just wiggle, then maybe I was okay. I thought I saw them wiggle. I signaled the nurse again.

"I've got an interview this morning; could you please call and cancel that? I have a dentist appointment this afternoon." There I was, still delegating and conducting business when it finally hit me: what if this is serious? I can't move! Am I paralyzed? What if I have to live the rest of my life in a wheelchair? And, God? If you're out there, didn't you know I was *trying*? I was out there *exercising*! And this is what I *get?!*

No more excuses

Two Asian nurses came in to put me on the x-ray table *and they couldn't lift me!* One even commented, "She's too heavy." And I thought, how did I

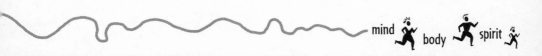

mind body spirit

let myself get like this? I wanted to tell them, wait, don't judge me, I really have been losing weight, I swear. That's why I was out there, after all, walking my weight off one day at a time.

As two male orderlies came in and lifted me, I cried. Not loud, wracking sobs that would have somehow been a relief, but silent tracks of tears out of the corners of my eyes, as I lay there for the world to see—fat, scared, vulnerable, embarrassed.

That's when I made the decision. I said, this is it, Tawni. You can use this as a line in the sand and be a victim again as usual—and no one would blame you. Or, as I reflected on all those choices in my life that inevitably came back to haunt me, what would your life be like if you chose something different? It's your choice.

I chose to believe—at that moment and for the rest of my moments on this earth—that I could rise above. I adopted a new mantra for myself: *No More Excuses!* In the cold, gray halls of the Seton emergency room, one of the obvious places where victimhood is excused, I chose not to be a victim.

In a place where people die routinely and without fanfare, lessons don't come easily. In fact, I have always found that in my life, the hard way is the only way. In the lesson at Seton Hospital, I found courage and strength I didn't even know I had. The will not just to survive, but to *thrive* overtook me and has powered my life ever since. In a way, I was blessed. My life had been spared. I needed to rise above the victim mentality. The day after the accident, I remember lying there in the hospital room, before anyone came—my sister or Martin, my boyfriend—thinking my life has a purpose or I would have been killed. I will see this through.

Why I'm here

A sense of purpose eluded me most of my life. Anyone looking through a crystal ball and following the path of my existence from the beginning would understand why. Even before I was born, I was unwanted. My parents were no more ready for me than for each other; it became literally an afterthought to get married.

Normally and ideally, two people come together, they love each other and they make the decision to have a family. This child is expected, welcomed, loved and nurtured from the time it is first placed in its mother's arms at the hospital. My parents' union was far from ideal and I never got that nurturing. What I found for myself instead was food.

Food was a natural solution. Cliched as it may sound, food for me was love. I sought and found the comfort I was missing from my family structure in ice cream, pizza, and cookies. And I got fat. Too fat to ever feel loved, but also too vulnerable to give up the only source of comfort I had ever known. It is a predicament that defined and constricted my life until that day in the Seton emergency room. There, my body broken, my spirit soared. And I realized I had found my purpose.

I know now that it is my purpose to give others what I never had, that they might be inspired to change their lives positively. The very thing that I never got may be the very thing I can give to people who struggle with themselves—inside and out—every day.

Back to my beginning

I was born in Los Angeles, CA, in a Salvation Army hospital for unwed mothers, finally pressed into the world by a mother whose trademark became constantly reminding me what a burden I was to her. I was even put up for adoption at one point, my mother wavering on the edge of being able to take care of me, but she and my father, Raymond (aka "Punky"), changed their minds (maybe because marriage seemed to present a solution). They were married one week later in Tijuana, Mexico, and it looked like there was at least some semblance of a family possible.

I have no real recollection of my father's face, although from pictures I saw later in my life, I seem to have inherited his dark skin and almost Hispanic features. A drummer in his own band, he wasn't around much. The two of them were separated more than they were together during my first nine years of life. The first two weren't that bad; they even had another child together, my sister, Tiffani. Perhaps they thought as so many people do that all they needed was some extra glue to stay attached. But I'm not talking about any fairy tale here. Neither of them was faithful.

Fate or whatever divine power rules this world had other ideas about the future. When my father was murdered during a restaurant robbery, I was nine years old. His family had a strange history of death. My father's sister choked on a jujube candy at 16 and died. His own father died from a heart attack, not so strange, but he was only 50.

Somehow I believe that I was more affected by his death than I knew. Or something was going on with me because around this time was also my first visit to a therapist. Social services, to be exact. My mother must have

mind ☀ body ☀ spirit ☀

thought she was being helpful. I don't remember much of what I talked about, but the trip to the ice cream store for hot fudge sundaes afterwards still sticks in my head.

My mother was a proud, hard-working woman who took her responsibility to me seriously if not willingly. With no financial support from my father yet never deigning to accept welfare, she took things into her own hands; she took two jobs and I was lucky if I saw her for two hours a day. Through notes my mother would leave me on the kitchen counter, I was able to pay bills, go to the post office, do the laundry and the grocery shopping. At nine, I grew up fast because I had to.

A different world

I think the strength and drive in my character comes from both my mother and a woman named Lois. My mother taught me my work ethic because she was a worker bee herself; I don't think she missed a day of work in her life and she's been with the same company the whole time.

Our grandparents, Lois and Fred lived in Ojai, CA. Until third grade, Tiffani and I lived there during the week and only came back to Oxnard, where my mother had moved us, on the weekends. The atmosphere at Lois and Fred's house, where we often spent time as children, was nurturing and warm. Lois baked cookies and loved to knit.

My sister craved this stable environment and stayed with Lois and Fred until she was old enough to be on her own. Even though being with Lois made me see that another world was possible, I think I felt this incredible loyalty to my mother and I stayed in her house as a child.

Looking back, I see Lois as a true blessing in my life. Reflecting on the positive things in my childhood, that is who I remember—meeting her at the end of her driveway, spending holidays together. We had chores and we learned discipline and good manners. If discipline was slow in coming, there was a wooden spoon or soap to wash out our mouths. I know that today people might call that child abuse, but then it was the best thing for me.

The "I Should" attitude

As an adult in my 20s, I whipped myself emotionally for not being able to handle what I thought would have been easy for my mother, whether it was a breakup or a professional challenge. To me, my mother was brave and strong.

No matter how many men she was involved with—and they were in and out of the house all the time, my so-called stepfathers—and no matter how many times a relationship went sour, she never showed weakness. I thought she was an emotional fortress and I tried to be just like her in that respect.

So began my "I should" attitude that stuck with me, for better or for worse (usually worse), all my life. The "I should" part of me meant that everything I did fell just short of good enough, that no matter how I tried, I could forget about measuring up—to my standards or anyone else's. I feel like it came less from anything my mother did and more as a punishment I doled generously out to myself.

Crawling into all areas of my life, I found that my "I should" attitude made any small goals that I would set for myself unacceptable. It was what I flayed myself with when I saw someone else do something I thought I should have been able to do myself. Although it did bring me success in terms of my career, it more significantly brought me sleepless nights and days of bingeing, packing those feelings of inadequacy in even more tightly.

The diet trap is set

One thing my mother clearly struggled with on a daily basis was her weight. She was always on one diet or another, trying hard to lose weight and the refrigerator reflected that. I never had sugar cereals in the house; diet coke, non-fat milk, sweet and low, those types of things were common, and fruits and vegetables. My mother never cooked. I remember making myself grilled cheese sandwiches and Campbell's tomato soup.

The concept of "diet" was obviously present from the start. My mother's battle with the bulge made me painfully aware of my own body image. But to me, food wasn't just nutrition. I needed something more, much more, and I took it from the Chase Brothers Dairy, stopping there on the way to junior high school. The cookies and ice cream that they sold me were my salvation, the only thing I could think of to make up for the loneliness of a mother who wasn't there. Of course I was busy with my chores around the house and my homework, but the food was my best friend, the one guaranteed to give me the solace I was looking for, however

> In the US, at least one child in five is overweight. Over the last two decades, the number of overweight children continues to grow, increasing by at least 50%. ...overweight children are at high risk of becoming overweight adolescents and adults.
>
> THE DAILY APPLE: YOUR EXPERT GUIDE TO DAILY HEALTH, AUGUST 1999

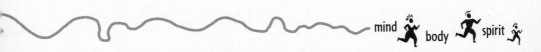

mind   body   spirit

temporary. I still missed having my mother there, having someone who would devote themselves to me and pay attention.

When I began to gain weight in 5th grade, that was something my mother noticed. After all, wasn't it me who was with her when she shopped at JC Penney, wore a size 14 and support pantyhose and complained about being too fat? She was always on a diet, so when I started to look a little flabby, she encouraged me to diet. I knew she understood my struggle, if only in terms of her own. Inside, though, I only lashed myself some more, tasting the bitter disappointment at letting myself *and* her down. I *should know* better, I silently screamed, because my own mother has the same problem.

In the United States, the food industry spends $36 billion a year on advertising, and much of it is aimed at children. The average American child sees 10,000 food advertisements each year on television alone. Ninety-five percent of those are for one of four types of foods, dense in calories and fat: fast foods, sugar-coated cereals, soft drinks or candy. And that's 10,000 messages by the brightest minds in advertising to convince children to eat foods that are bad for them.

PROF. KELLY BROWNELL, DIR. YALE CENTER FOR EATING AND WEIGHT DISORDERS ON FRONTLINE, 11/3/98

My mother couldn't understand how I was gaining weight. I guess she must have thought my entrance into puberty was simply marked by a few extra pounds. I understood all too well. Not only was I sneaking food all the time but hiding my eating was my master illusion. The trick was not eating in front of people when I was going to eat a lot. It's a habit that I still carry with me today; I try hard not to eat in public. Plus we had just moved again, away from friends I used to spend afternoons roller skating with and the school I knew, to a nicer place where I felt more alone than ever. My mom continued to work all the time and the only company I would have during the day was her second husband, a professional piano player.

One day I was sitting at the piano (his) with him, on his lap, and he was supposedly showing me something on the keyboard. He was often home during the day because he played at night. While he did this, he moved me around (to get himself off, I now know). I remember thinking, quit poking me, but I didn't think much of it at the time.

Then came the night he went into my bedroom. I had a canopy bed and the frills that you would expect in a girl's room: pink and white of course. He had his boxer shorts on and he climbed into bed with me, claiming he was going to keep me company until my mother came home. The company he kept meant kissing and fondling me and taking my panties off.

On one level, it felt good. I mean, there I was, a young girl, and a man was paying attention to me. I thought, this is love; someone is loving me. I didn't know that sex wasn't love because sex was all I had been shown when I grew up. After all, there were always men around the house. My mother seemed to go from man to man and marriage to marriage just like changing underwear. I even remember hearing my mother having sex with whatever man she was involved with or married to.

The next morning, I felt strange and I knew it was wrong. From then on, when I came home from school, I went into my bedroom and locked the door. I locked the door at night, too.

More importantly, I remember having food in my bedroom with me, hiding it under my bed. I would have done anything not to be in his presence. I had a television and a phone, so I sat in my room, did homework, watched Charlie's Angels—and I ate.

You didn't protect me!

Although I have been able to at least come to terms with this early abuse later, all I could feel at the time was anger. As an adult, I remember telling only one therapist about the sexual molestation. And I didn't want to break up the marriage; somewhere in my mind, I was thinking, "I don't want to bother anyone or cause any chaos."

But I resented my mother. Even though she was lonely, and in some respects a party girl who liked company, she was also the one person in the world who was supposed to protect me and all she did was bring more and more men into the house who ended up hurting me.

Logically, I realized that my mother was only trying to raise me the best way she knew how. No one gave her any lessons. Emotionally, it wasn't that easy to accept. In a way, my relationships with men mirrored what I had always yearned for with my mother. Because I grew up feeling like I was a bother and always in the way, that just the mere fact of existing had ruined my mother's life, as an adult, I craved attention and affection, someone who would spend time with me.

I was instead attracted to men who were successful yet had little or no time for me. Of course this was only natural because it was the most famil-

mind body spirit

iar to me. As a child I felt my mother had no time for me and I still feel this way today. That core of nurturing love that kids around me grew up taking for granted—and sometimes even resisting—was sorely missing for me. Instead it seemed like every time my mother took an action, it just created chaos for my world.

Alone at Grandma's

When I was in 5th grade, the piano player was scheduled to play a gig on a cruise ship and at the last minute, my mother decided to go along. So she drove me over to my grandmother's house (Freda, her mom) and dropped me off. My grandma Freda wasn't home at the time, but I remember my mother convinced me that she would be back and would take care of me.

Well, unknown to her, my grandmother had left for the weekend, so I was alone in the house until my mother returned a few days later. I remember being really afraid and telling myself I had to be strong. Instead I stuffed everything I could find in the cabinets and cupboards of the house into my scared ten-year-old body.

I didn't know when anyone was going to come and get me and once again it was more important for my mother to take that cruise than to take care of me and make sure that I wasn't alone. So I ate out of fear and I ate out of anger toward my mom.

The loudest voice on earth

At five feet tall and 140 pounds, with a tin smile and acne rearing its unwelcome head, I suffered every day I went to junior high school. As luck would have it, I even suffered the excruciating embarrassment of a teacher's aid shouting my weight over to another person who recorded it for my school file. I thought, great, glad you told that to everyone! I didn't need the reminder; I had my own voice inside my own head to shout it every day.

I had just gotten off the scale, the kind that clanks when you move the notch over, and that really made it glaring. No one reacted or said anything to me, but they didn't have to. The chant inside my head ran something like "I'm fatter than everyone else." And it was true! Everyone else in 7th grade weighed 90 or 95 pounds. I weighed as much as my mother! I was really fat.

I had no refuge at school or at home. The only thing I could do was to eat over everything. It wasn't even a conscious decision at that point. Whatever crisis arose in my young life, I stopped up my flow of feelings with food like you would cork a bottle.

Every time my mother decided to remarry (a lot of times), that meant we moved. To comfort myself during these times of upheaval, I stole money from my mother's wallet to support my ice cream habit. Or a hamburger joint would open up nearby and I would buy ice cream cones dipped in chocolate. It was the closest I could get to paradise, every sugary mouthful a balm on my wounded self.

During the summer after junior high, my mother sent me to a "fat farm," cleverly disguised as a camp. It was here that I ran for the first time and saw what exercise could do for me. I lost 35 pounds and was thin for the first time.

When I started high school, finished with braces, with a new body and the prospect of new friends on the horizon, I was jubilant. No one had to know I used to be fat. I even joined the cross country team. I thought running would keep me thin and I didn't think I had the coordination for any other sports.

Although I loved being part of a team, I hated running. Running took discipline. We ran five days a week and as many as ten miles a day,

> "...bulimia is an addiction that's hard to break. It requires enormous willpower to fight the urge to binge and purge. And unlike people with other addictions such as alcohol or cocaine, bulimic women can't avoid their drug of choice...Fighting the urge to binge is just one part of the treatment. [You also need] new ways to deal with...psychic pain. Bulimia, like all addictions, is a way to run from pain."
>
> MARY PIPHER, PHD. FROM REVIVING OPHELIA

between distance work and mile repeats. And it was *hard!* I was one of the slowest runners on the team, but my sheer paranoia of being again, my utter fear of returning to an older version of my body, kept me going. I never felt fast or even that I was a good runner, but I did feel like I was an athlete, especially since we got to wear uniforms and I was in shape.

There was a street in Camarillo, CA called Fairview. It was in the hilly estate area and it went up, up, up. Well, one day I decided I would tackle that road and wearing my white dolphin shorts and a blue shirt, I plowed right up. I remember being inwardly triumphant, and thinking, hot damn, I'm in good shape! I mean, my *car* couldn't even get up this hill. I was really proud of myself for running every day and doing my best.

I also ran in races. Of course I was always in the back working my way forward, but I plugged along. I was even given the award by the team for being the "most inspirational." Even if I weren't setting speed records or

mind 🏃 body 🏃 spirit 🏃

bringing back first place trophies, I glowed with the knowledge that I could be useful to others, that people seemed to need my encouraging words.

Another thing running brought me was a hero. Two years older than me, Vivian was tall and thin, a typical runner, with brown hair and olive skin. She was even smart, graduating as the valedictorian of her class. I think she ended up going to Stanford. I idolized her running and her brain. Vivian won almost every race she entered. Happily she was supportive and encouraging to me. I remember running around the track doing mile repeats and even though Vivian would pass me again and again, she would call out encouragement each time she ran by. Every now and then, I still hear her cheers.

Still battling the almighty calorie

Running all those miles during cross-country practice yet still having to count calories and watch my weight upset me. It wasn't fair! Even though I was fitting into sizes 5 and 7 clothing, I had days where I would binge and turn all this hatred against myself. I would tell myself, I feel too fat to run after school today. The running was hard—the excuses were easy.

During the week, I was too busy with school and running to have time to eat. The weekends became my time to release all that control—and I did. Whole, giant-sized bags of Fritos, entire half gallons of ice cream, whole pizzas meant to feed four people—all that and more fell before me. Afterwards, empty containers with the last remains of crusts or chip dust or sticky ice cream residue would be strewn on the bed and the floor, and I would lie on my bed and think, I can't believe I ate all that. It was all about filling up and eating fast. I still eat fast and I have to consciously slow myself down.

Those binge days led me to treat my body and my self even more poorly. I had to do something to correct those out of control episodes. I don't know whether it was in the media or some of the other girls were talking about it, but bulimia seemed like the perfect solution. I discovered bulimia as though finding a long-lost companion to my eating.

At the time, I was living in a little studio add-on to the house with a kitchen and a bathroom. But even though it was easy for me to live without hiding things, I would still bury all the evidence of my eating in the bottom of the trash can. Then I would go throw up, as if it were as normal as brushing my teeth. I never told anyone; it just became my dirty little secret. It was always a relief, too, because during the week I had had to tell myself "no, no, Tawni" when I wanted to eat something I liked. Finally the weekend would arrive and I could eat all I wanted. Going in circles, I didn't do it every day, but I did continue all through high school, running and throwing up whenever I perceived I ate too much or the wrong things.

Combining bulimia with laxatives, I was able to achieve the instant gratification that food had become for me and still feel like I wouldn't pay the price for eating. And because I wanted to keep eating that way, I kept running and started being bulimic to stave off this horrible crawling fear of gaining weight.

I managed to stay thin the whole four years doing this, until my senior year when I injured my right knee. Maybe it was just runner's knee, but it was bad enough to prevent me from running. I tried to keep running, but it hurt, and the pounding of my feet changed into the drumbeat of my fears: Oh my God, I'm going to get fat. Because not running changed all my patterns and my binges were no longer confined to the weekends.

Our choices have consequences and back then I didn't want the consequences. But in this case, the consequences were inevitable. Before I knew it, I had gained 20 pounds in two months. It was an injury I would carry with me for the next few years, but at the time, all I could think about was that I wouldn't be able to fit into my senior prom dress, a peach colored garment left over from a wedding my mother had attended. I was supposed to attend my senior prom with a guy named Steve. A whole group of us were renting a limousine and it was supposed to be the usual big affair that a prom is in high school.

I went to try on the dress and it was *tight!* I was horrified. While I wasn't *huge,* I was disgusted with myself. I was working at Miller's Outpost at the time and when I got off work at nine at night, I ran in spite of the excruciating pain in my knee. After a month of running, the night of the prom arrived and the dress didn't fit any better than it had before.

In desperation, I found one of my grandmother's corsets and I wore that under the dress. I spent the whole night uncomfortable and strapped into that contraption. When we went out for dinner, I didn't even eat because there wasn't a spare inch in that dress! No one suspected, but I knew, and I was ashamed.

mind body spirit

Money for friendship

During my late teens and early twenties, my sole focus was on college. I thought that if could just get through my classes, not gain any more weight and find the man of my dreams, my problems would be over. I had no real thoughts of my future; I only lived in this weird world made up of my weight, my studies and my attempts to make friends.

I did find that I wanted to be with people. Somehow I was more at ease when I was not alone and as an adult I can see that I was craving what I never had as a child: companionship, attention, love. And self-worth? I had little or none. The only way I saw that people would want to be with me was for me to buy them. I invited people to lunch—and paid. I took them shopping—and bought them expensive gifts. If I was dating a guy, besides throwing myself into a massive round of dieting, I would buy him lavish presents. Generally, my attitude was that if I bought people things, they would like me.

I had money because after my father's murder, I received social security benefits. I first used that money for a new car when I was 16 and monthly car payments led to tons of credit card offers. And I bought stuff not for myself, but for others. I just wanted someone to go with me. If it was a trip I wanted to go on, I'd invite someone and pay for them. How could someone refuse that kind of offer? In the end, I think it came down to my fear of people not accepting me the way I was: insecure, overweight, fearful.

But this freewheeling spending spree had to end somewhere. The credit cards that were so easy to get weren't as simple to pay off. I made the choice to use money to buy people—including and especially men. As a result, I spent my entire twenties in credit card debt. Even now, the money I have in the bank calls my name, just like the food always has. It takes as much of my willpower not to head out for Nordstrom's as it does not to head for Dairy Queen.

Hitting the relationship wall

College found me working part time and going to school full time. A hard road of lessons lay ahead of me, although I didn't know it at the time. When I first moved out of my mother's house, all I thought about was the freedom. When I lived with my mother, my room was always perfect, my grades were always perfect, and I was the perfect "wife" to her. Finally I could have men over to my apartment any time I want. I could come and go all I want. Funny, though, I still had these weird food issues. I would order pizza and then take my trash out to the big dumpster, so no one, not even me, would know I had been eating it. Big time shame.

It didn't take long for me to hit an emotional wall. As a freshman in college, I started dating a good-looking man in his early twenties named Ray who had already finished college. Ray was my older fantasy, my picture of an ideal. I had my own place, he had his—it was a "grownup" relationship. We worked out at a gym together, and I was doing pretty well with my weight again. In fact, we did all kinds of activities: low-impact aerobics, biking, hiking, weights, etc. I had my first sexual experience (with someone I wanted to be with) with Ray. My bulimia had tapered off. Things could not have been better.

One day, after I had lunch with Ray, I decided to visit his best friend's girlfriend who worked at a hair salon in the nearby shopping mall. I had just gotten over having strep throat and I was anxious to see people again. As I was sitting in a chair in the beauty salon, reflected in the mirrors on the wall, I saw the man who was supposed to be my boyfriend holding hands with another girl.

I sprang out of my seat and walked over to him, only to have the further humiliation of Ray introducing me to this girl—her name was Linda and they ended up getting married—like it was the most normal thing in the world. What could I say? This girl obviously knew nothing of me. I walked away and was physically sick in a mall bathroom. That was just the beginning.

The suffering ran through my body and my heart. I couldn't make myself believe it. I felt so taken. All that ran through my simple 19 year old head was, "But I just had lunch with you!" So that was it. My world, revolving in all its simplicity around Ray, had shattered. As far as I was concerned, my life was over. Here was a love that I thought would last forever and now just look how easy it was for him to end it.

I spent a miserable night alone in my apartment, sleepless and crying until I was exhausted. I couldn't see how my life would ever be better again. And there was the unspoken but haunting chant inside of me: "I'm not good enough." So I got in my car the next morning and drove to the drugstore where I bought two bottles of sleeping pills. To me this would be easy; I would just take the pills and go to sleep and it would all be over. How nice that sounded to my aching heart.

mind body spirit

Of course, all I really performed was a half-hearted show of bravado. A handful of pills and I woke up the next morning, completely discouraged from waking up. But after I slept off the effects of the pills and the sun still insisted on shining through my window, I thought, "okay, I didn't die, so there must be a reason."

Now I was angry. How dare he! Looking for a fast, maybe easy way to get past this betrayal, I packed Ray's things that were in my apartment. Sneaking over to his place, I put the box in his car, thinking that was the end of it. Not quite!

Not only did I have the picture of them together in my head, I also had my own voice telling me I should be stronger, I should be able to handle this, and so on. I couldn't. I dropped out of college for a year, unable to face even the most mundane tasks.

Even worse, I had no support from my mother. She was unapproachable, busy as she was running her own life, and told me to pull myself together. What's the big deal, she asked. It's just a man. So again I was hit with the unattainable goal of "I should." Why wasn't I braver? How could she be so strong all the time? Why didn't I have a higher regard for myself than to let a man make me feel so rotten about myself?

I didn't get over Ray for quite a while. I missed him and the betrayal created a huge trust issue that pursued me through all the relationships I have had since. No matter how good I feel about a relationship I am in, there is still that nagging knowledge that there are no guarantees. I find myself wondering, will this one *really* stay with me? Does he *really* love me the way he says he does?

Throughout my twenties, I let destructive relationships with men overtake me. Any man that paid attention to me was my sole criteria for sex. Married, single, girlfriends or not, all I cared about was getting next to a warm body. It was a downward spiral of bars and nightclubs, alcohol and abuse, and more than one scary experience I didn't know if I would walk away from.

And despite being responsible and using condoms most of the time, I still managed to get pregnant. It didn't seem like a big deal to me at the time. I remember thinking, "well, I'm pregnant and I don't want the kid," so I just dealt with it. But it became one more thing piled on top of the rest of it all. Now I was a bad girl who had done a bad thing. Worse, the only thing I felt guilty about was not feeling guilty about the abortion.

I could whine and say that it wasn't my fault. In fact, I did. But looking back, I know I had choices and I didn't make the right ones.

My attitude about sex was worst of all. Struggling with my weight as I did, I felt like I was lucky that *any* man would want to be that close to me. And when I didn't feel like having sex, I had it anyway. I remember my mom telling me, sex is not worth arguing about and it's over with so fast anyway. So I didn't argue; I just said, okay, I'll have sex with you, even if I didn't want to.

You can see a picture of me during those times—a lonely, needy girl searching for who she was as a woman, fighting a body she hated, missing the nurturing a mother had no time to give.

My own pattern of promiscuity followed in turn. I looked for happiness and acceptance from creatures of the male persuasion, but found very little, actually. The only true friend, the only constant and unfailing companion, was food. And to this I devoted myself. Some kids had imaginary friends; I had food. And the best part was no one had to know. Through all my closet eating, my bulimia, etc., it was my secret.

Secrecy always the key

Another secret I kept in my mid-20s was alcohol. My parents were alcoholics and so were my grandparents. It would have been easy for me to become yet another statistic. I would drink alone in my apartment, sometimes to numb this inexplicable pain inside, sometimes just to go to sleep. I never drank in public; I didn't want to lose control. Telling myself I drank out of depression made it seem like I was more in control. There was no hiding the fact that, just like when I ate, I had not just one drink, but the whole blender full.

Luckily, I recognized the behavior. And even more luckily, it scared me. A therapist I was seeing recommended that I go to Alcoholics Anonymous. I really believe in having support and in that sense, the group sessions were helpful. Of course, I didn't really think I was that bad, I didn't see myself as one of the others—losing their jobs, their homes, their families over alcohol. What I could relate to was the compulsiveness, the drinking to forget, the drinking to numb the loneliness and depression. That I understood. I always had. And I learned to stop drinking.

mind body spirit

Nevertheless, I became and remained a secretive adult. I used the food as my shield. I was always nervous meeting new people and tried to make some excuse to avoid it. Maybe that was because I was constantly searching for acceptance and love from other people, yet I was never quite sure that anyone would actually *want* to be close to me—whether it was a friendship or a relationship.

Desperate for a solution to my whirlwind of issues, I spent much of my twenties in therapy with social workers, mental health therapists, etc. I had to come to terms with so much and be able to carry on in the face of my attitude that the world would be better off without me. In essence, I paid someone to listen to me because I didn't want to bother anyone I knew with my stuff. I tried as many anti-depressants as therapists, bouncing on and off Prozac, Zoloft, or Paxil like some rubber ball bouncing from ceiling to floor.

Three years of my late twenties found me on and off all these different anti-depressants, and the whole time I felt awful, drugged, had terrible headaches and was unable to think clearly. If I felt like I was on an emotional roller coaster, the doctors would try to level me out and there were more side effects. I got to the point that I didn't know which emotions were mine and which were the drugs'. Worst of all, some drugs made me sick to my stomach while others compelled me to eat even more. I finally separated myself from what I now see as a crutch that doesn't work—or at least not for me—and at the very least doesn't solve the real inner problems.

After college, I worked for my mother's company in customer service and later at other companies in outside sales. In my work, when people reached out to me, I requested to be transferred to a different department. Ironic, isn't it? All my life I just wanted people to like me, yet I put on a literal barrier to keep them at arm's length. I think I must have been convinced that on some level, if I did respond to people who reached out to me, that I would be scorned in the end. I was afraid that they would discover all my secrets and reject the person I was. I couldn't trust that anyone would like me for me.

But I couldn't go on that way forever. I couldn't want intimacy and at the same time continue to reject it. On a deeper level, I always wanted to matter. I wanted to give love and receive it in return. With my mother, I wanted to make it worth her effort in bringing me into this world. With men, I needed to feel secure within myself so I could feel secure with them. As far as my body and soul, there had to come a point when I said to myself, Tawni, you really *do* have to change your life. You really *aren't* healthy, you *aren't* living in reality, and the changes have to be inside *and* out.

CHAPTER 2

Lifestyle change

I think I'm finally grasping the fact that there is no finish line. I must constantly change the way I used to think if I'm going to continue to be successful at this thing called life. It's through making better choices about what goes into my body everyday that I'm starting to see how it's all 'connected.' By making myself a priority, I'm starting to feel like I matter. And the person I matter most to is me!

I'm slowly learning to set boundaries and make better choices for me. It takes such COURAGE to make different choices. It's easier to go with the flow. I pray for COURAGE everyday.

JOURNAL ENTRY, JULY 9, 1997

M aking a commitment to a lifestyle change is not just a one-time deal: it's minute by minute and day by day. And there will be moments that you feel the demons of temptation crawling toward you. You'll have days where the only place you can find discipline is in the dictionary.

It's during these times that you will be powered by your core motivation for changing your life. So before you ever run two feet or bike one mile, decide what that motivation is for you. Because it's not just about changing your physical self; it's about transforming mentally and spiritually. You could be the thinnest person in the world and not be happy. So it's not just the body; it's everything connected together.

Don't underestimate the power of a decision. When I took hold of myself at Seton Hospital, I really grasped that decision and I have never looked back. That's not to say that I don't have bad days and make bad food choices. I do. But I feel better about the majority of the choices that I make. And it shows—both physically and mentally.

What compelled me to change

I don't believe that in life there is ever really one single factor that makes you change. Instead, it is usually a combination of things, a cumulative effect, built-up frustration or just plain getting sick of your lifestyle.

Like so many other women who have tried to lose weight—through diets, books, pills—I have tried just about everything. I Weight Watch-ed, Jenny Craig-ed, Slim Fast-ed and Nutri-system-ed. I read Susan Powter's

mind body spirit

book, but I didn't really relate to her. I bought just about every new diet book that came on the market, thinking, this time for sure, this is the one that will make me turn my life around.

In my mid to late twenties, I attended Overeater's Anonymous (OA) for about two years and worked my way through the 12 steps. That was progress for me especially since I had been berating myself: Tawni, you're getting older and this is ridiculous. You can't keep living like there's no tomorrow. I had to take personal inventory and that was helpful in taking responsibility and not continuing to heap easy blame on my childhood for my adult problems. I began to let go of the victim role that I had been using to get myself attention for so long and that was cleansing. I think I lost some weight, but OA helped me more psychologically than physically.

In the spring 1994, I was living in Ventura when the company I was working for offered me a job in San Francisco. With no place to live, I decided to go for it. I was looking for an escape, feeling like I had to get the hell out of southern California. I had met Martin, my husband, at a leadership seminar and happened to mention that I was moving to San Francisco. He offered to help me move and I accepted his offer.

In November 1994, I rented a 26-foot U-Haul truck and packed up my two bedroom house. With Martin's 1991 blue Mustang on a trailer behind the U-Haul, he took charge of the huge rig and I followed him in my car. We left on a Friday night and headed up Highway 101. We reached a Best Western in South San Francisco later that evening. We spent the next day searching for a place for me to live. When we returned to the hotel, we noticed that the lock had been broken off the back of the U-Haul and some stuff had been taken.

After filing a police report, the police officer suggested that we park the U-Haul in front of a nearby restaurant because not only were people in and out of it all the time, but apparently it was a police hangout as well.

It was early evening and both of us went out to the U-Haul to get some clothes for the next day. Out of nowhere, four men approached us. They hardly said a word to us, but the attitude was, okay, we're taking your stuff. They spoke to each other, as if we weren't there: "get in the truck," "tie them up." Martin and I were just in shock. I was absolutely paralyzed.

Tied together with rope and thrown on the ground, I watched as they hotwired the U-Haul and drove away with all my worldly belongings, but not before one of them walked up and whacked me over the head with his pistol.

In the course of ten minutes, my life had been completely pulled out from under me. I cried until I was sick to my stomach from crying. When someone from the hotel found us, I tried to be composed—both for the hotel front desk and for the police, with whom I once again filed a report. I thought, I have to contain myself. And I couldn't. I called my boss, told him everything I owned had been stolen and what do I do?

I ended up living with my boss for a month. People at my new job donated things to me, like napkins, silverware, chairs, and clothes. Martin flew back to Los Angeles, but promptly sent me his credit card by Federal Express, telling me I could pay him back when I was able to.

I was miserable. It rained every day I was there. I thought, moving here is the worst mistake I have ever made. But even though I felt the odds were against me and my mother was encouraging me to come back to southern California, I decided that I might as well make a go of this. Even if I moved back, I would still have to buy new things.

Martin flew up every weekend to help me. Finally, my boss offered him a job and he was able to move to San Francisco a few months later. But starting out, I was absolutely despondent.

There I was, all alone in a new city, with all my things gone, getting lost every time I tried to go anywhere. I hated the weather. I was working like a maniac and having to spend any money that I made on clothes and furniture. At first all I had was a cardboard box for a table and I slept on the floor. And worse, these were the holidays and my birthday, too. I was flooded with all these memories from the past of where I spent holidays, especially of Grandma Lois.

So what did I do? I ate. Domino's pizza was on my speed dial. I ordered food in because it was easier. I didn't have to go out and find some place to eat. Hot pepperoni pizza with extra cheese and ahhh. That made it a little better. And chocolate chip ice cream—or cookies and cream, depending on my mood. Or maybe both. I was so depressed and so immersed in the victim role that I was so good at. Poor me. Look at what has happened to me now. From November 1994 to January 1996, I gained 90 pounds, blowing up to my highest weight ever: 275 pounds.

When I had decided to make the move to San Francisco, running from southern California like a scared little rabbit, I felt like a new city would be a fresh start for me. Reflecting on my feelings during that time, I know what I felt was tired. I felt like a big failure because I knew better but I couldn't

mind body spirit

stop eating anyway. I got to the point where I just said, "I don't care. I give up. I'm tired of trying to be strong."

So I just continued to balloon. Work was great, though. Of course! It was the one thing I knew I was good at. Spring 1995 found me at one of Tony Robbins' seminars. I was constantly attending these; since I was in sales, it was a normal thing to do. But the difference here was that it was like adding another drop of water into the bucket that represented me making a change. I thought, I'm wasting my potential. Why should I only be successful in one area of my life? Why should I let the past continue to literally eat away at me?

I could relate so well to some of the things that Tony Robbins said. I read all of his books and I remembered his statement that the past doesn't equal the future. That made so much sense to me because I was always living in the past, beating myself up for my own life and the choices I had made in it. He also said that at any given moment you can change. When I read that, it gave me hope. Even though I wasn't quite ready to make that change, I was close.

By spring 1995, I was also finally taking responsibility for my problem with men, too. Before I was just manipulative and deceiving in any way to get what I wanted from a man. If I wanted to see some guy, I would just say, oh I'm going to be in the neighborhood on a certain day and we would do lunch, even if in reality I had to drive two hours out of my way to meet him.

In January 1996, I made a New Year's resolution to finally lose weight. This was a time I also joined Weight Watchers, which helped if I followed the program. I tried to exercise, too. Without any set plan, I was just doing a little walking here and there. Nothing consistent. My eating habits hadn't changed; I was still devouring tons of fast food, especially Taco Bell.

I didn't get in gear until September 1996.

On a trip to Phoenix, AZ, I was holed up in a hotel room, grabbing a quick bite (literally—I think it was Burger King) and catching the Oprah Show. As she came on stage, it was obvious that she was jubilant. Oprah looked wonderful and she radiated this glowing confidence through and through. I remember this chaotic mix of emotions inside of me. As always, there was the lashing, punishing voice of guilt: Tawni, you are no good. You're fat and no one will ever love you the way you are.

Then there was this other voice, one I hadn't heard before: Tawni, if Oprah can do it, so can you. Whoa! Was that a new one! It felt good, really good. Of course, it had a companion on its heels: "What are you, crazy, Tawni? Oprah did it with a trainer. She had someone to help her. You can't do it alone." And I thought, "wrong. I can do it because all that I need to do it is already inside of me. I can do it because it is the best thing I can do not just for my body, but also for my head. After all, there is only room for one voice in there and I get to choose which one it is!"

In that moment, the urge to make a change became larger than it had ever been for me before. I knew that I could make the decision to change, but I was afraid. I was afraid to fail, I was afraid that I would just end up disappointing myself one more time. I mean, I went through a lot of times where I promised myself I would do something. I would go on one diet or another, always with the hope that my solution, my salvation in the form of weight loss, would come easily and quickly. Boy was I not living in reality.

I went out and bought Oprah's book, *Make the Connection* and read it, just as I had read all the others. I approached it as just another diet. I didn't know that it would be the final link in the chain of events I had needed to change my life.

Until my accident in December 1996, I think that somewhere, deep down, I figured I would probably give up the Oprah-related routine, too, at some point. How could I take my attempt to change seriously when this was just more of the same thing I had done before?

Instead my impulse became routine. Where before there were empty words, now I took action. Just like being in sales, I started setting realistic goals and saw the real possibility of achieving them, instead of starting out with the broad (and mostly fruitless) plan to lose weight.

I realized that I had always been searching for the answers outside of myself. Finally I reached a point where I could see that it is *my* choice in everything that affects what I do, how I act, what I look like, where I go in life, etc. Even though I still battle excuses, it is powerful to make choices and accept responsibility for those choices, knowing deep down that those choices are now the best ones I can make at the time and not ones I will regret later.

Until a few years ago, I lived my life trying to please other people. People I worked with and met on a daily basis only knew me as successful, smart, and hard-working. They didn't know my other side. Of course they never commented on my being fat; they were too polite. I never reached a level of real honesty all my life with people or men because I was too busy being

mind body spirit

what I thought they wanted me to be. I thought that was what would make people love me. I thought that if they knew who I really was, where I had been, what I had gone through—they wouldn't like the real Tawni.

What I learned is that to give to others and stay healthy doing it, you have to give to yourself first. Making a lifestyle change has made me better able to give to people, to give of my *self* in the way that I want. I have also come to the (late) conclusion that perfection is impossible. Sounds like common sense, but it really wasn't for me for a long time. I still go through these times when I think, things will be perfect if I just control them. I recognize my tendency to want to control things and now I can just be with it. I acknowledge those feelings instead of repressing—stuffing myself, literally—with them.

And while I have done a lot of growing up, I'm not done; I'm not at the end of my journey. I still have "stuff" to fix, weight to lose, issues to keep addressing. What I have learned is that change can be positive, no matter how much challenge you have to go through first to get to the changing part.

So the "big picture" answer is that my changes made me want to help others change. I have started to see how my life has turned around for the better and now I wanted to reach out and share that experience. I *know* how hard it is to change. I have been there. I *know* the fear of failure. I *know* the voice of guilt. I want to share what I have learned so that if you decide to make a lifestyle change for yourself, I can make it that much easier.

Oprah's Connection

When I first read Bob Greene and Oprah's book, *Make the Connection*, I was looking for anything to latch onto to give me some direction, some focus to make a change in my life. I instinctively knew that what I was about to embark upon would affect all areas in my life: my body, my mind, my soul, my lifestyle, my relationships, my work, everything.

What I found was what Bob and Oprah call their "ten steps to a better body—and a better life" which I immediately decided to adopt for my own life. These ten steps eventually became my steps of "training for life." Now, I have taken their steps and modified them slightly, and even annotated them. But I am enormously grateful to Bob and Oprah, and acknowledge them for giving me the guidance I needed to get started. Here is my version of ten steps to changing your life:

1 **Exercise aerobically, preferably six days each week.** But this does not mean you have to do exactly the same type of exercise every day (e.g., cross-train running with cycling, or walking with water fitness, etc.)

2 **Exercise at a level that makes you sweat and during which you can just barely talk aloud comfortably.** Bob Greene likes calling this level "the zone." It's knowing when you are pushing yourself, but not overdoing it.

3 **Exercise at least 30 minutes or more, preferably more for each workout.** Given that it takes at least 10 minutes to just get warmed up metabolically, why work out less than this except when you are just starting out. If you are new to exercise, its okay to try to strive for maybe 20 minutes until you become better conditioned aerobically. Then you can go for as long as you can. I now work out for the better part of an hour (sometimes longer on some days) nearly every day.

4 **Eat a low-fat, balanced diet each day.** Balanced means from the traditional four food groups. And this does not mean a cheeseburger (breads & cereals, and meats), fries (fruits & vegetables), and a shake (dairy products) either.

5 **Eat several meals a day, including low-fat snacks, but try to eat most of your food early on in the day.**

6 **Don't drink alcohol.** I am a recovering alcoholic, so this is not an option.

7 **Stop eating two to three hours before going to bed.** This is difficult for most people because of the temptation to snack while watching TV or whatever.

8 **Drink up to eight glasses of water a day.** This can be hard to do because water is so boring. I would much rather drink a six-pack of Pepsi.

9 **Eat two servings of fruit and three servings of vegetables each day** (e.g., an apple is one serving, a cup of orange juice is also one serving of fruit).

10 **Stay focused each day by recommitting yourself to a healthy body and mind.**

I must admit that there are times that following all ten of these steps each day can be difficult. I mean, sometimes I can't find any decent fruit to eat. Or perhaps I'm traveling and I can't work out on a day that I would normally work out (although I usually make sure I make up for a lost day on another day, no excuses). Or sometimes I don't drink as much water as I should. And so on. But generally I am consistent. And consistency is important.

You can't just decide to be a part-time fitness- and health-conscious person. There is no such thing. It's like the fair weather runners I see. When it's raining, or cold, or unusually windy, I never see these people. But when it's the weekend, and the sun is out, and the temperature is nice, and the sky is blue and beautiful, all of a sudden, it seems everyone in the world has become a runner or a walker.

By not being consistent, by not working out no matter what the conditions—even in rain, hail, sleet, or snow—you may as well not waste your time working out at all. Working out occasionally will not significantly change your life. This also applies to all other areas of your life. By not being consistent in your food choices, or how much water you drink, or how often and when you eat, you will not make a significant change in your life. I'm not just talking about losing weight, I'm talking about a mind, body, and soul change. This is something that must start from within to have an effect on all aspects of your life.

Starting the Connectors

In September 1996, I posted a message on the Oprah.com boards in the "100 pounds or more" to lose folder. I asked, has anyone read *Make the Connection* and is there a support group? The people who posted replies to me responded that there wasn't, and these were the first few people I started writing to and encouraging in their journey.

I started by sending out a thought for the day, reflecting on the difficulties and offering hope for the future. I would often issue a challenge. For instance, I had a big Pepsi addiction, so one of my challenges was I'm only going to drink four diet Pepsis today and one glass of water; anyone else?

A group of about 100 of us held together for about three years that way, taking the bumps and potholes on the weight loss road in stride, strong because of our common connection and mutual struggles.

I started the Connectors Web site in January 1999 after I approached *Runner's World* to do a story on the Connectors that would run in February 1999. I knew that *Runner's World* had a huge circulation and I wanted to give people a place to go.

At this point, the Connectors were moving beyond just simple support and weight loss. We were training for marathons and smaller runs. More and more often, people were posting messages and sending me emails excitedly reporting that they had just finished a 5k race. Even if they had half-walked, half-run the three miles, with knees hurting or side aches bending them in two, they had *finished!*

Before the Portland, OR Marathon in October 1998, I was ready to stop the emails. Despite the reports of victories, I felt like I wasn't getting that much out of it. I felt like I was doing all the giving; they all loved getting my thought for the day, but I was spending a tremendous amount of time each day responding to emails. It was too much, especially for someone who had just started a new job.

I think running that marathon and being with all those Connectors was what made me realize that people were counting on me. As the numbers of emails I received each day started to skyrocket, I reached down inside of myself and knew that I had to lead. They were my reason to keep going. They inspired me. I understood then that that was their gift to me: giving and receiving love.

Making your own choice

No one can make the decision to change your life but you. You can read my story and see parallels with your own life—you might even be inspired by it—but my story isn't yours. You have to write your own story, and to do that, you have to make the choice, make the commitment, and follow through with the action. It's not easy. Sometimes you'll feel as if everything and everyone in the world are working against you. Those are the times when it's easy to give up and easy to justify giving up. That certainly was my habit—to fall back on being a victim when the going got tough and to tell myself that I just couldn't fight such enormous odds.

When you're *really* ready to make the choice to change your life, you can overcome anything. But understanding your patterns, understanding how you use fat, knowing what you're facing before you begin, and throwing out all those self-defeating attitudes will give you that much more of a head start on success.

There are many reasons *not* to change your life, and the pressures of what you see around you in our society today don't help. You are always being given some excuse to latch on to personally or commercially.

Ways you use fat
Control

Fat can make you feel like you are out of control. You can use this as an excuse for not doing anything, either daily or overall in your life.

What does this mean? For me it meant that I never went to the beach. I wouldn't wear shorts. I wouldn't meet people because I was embarrassed

mind   body   spirit

at how I looked. I would be conveniently busy. If people were making plans for the weekend, I would say I already had plans. If a group of people wanted to go out after work, I would tell them I had too much work, but that I might join them later. Of course I didn't. Fat kept me on the sidelines.

After the U-Haul incident, I was gaining so much weight so fast, it was obvious I was out of control. It became a vicious cycle of making money combined with "hand to mouth." This was an emotional crisis! I thought, now I need to eat more than ever, so just leave me alone. I just had everything stolen from me, so I wasn't going to deny myself anything else. This was about deprivation versus abundance. I was only focused on what life was lacking. I knew better in a logical way, but I didn't care. It was like, so what? I didn't want anyone to tell me differently.

I alternated pizza places so the delivery guy wouldn't see that he was delivering to me every day. I'd eat and eat and eat, getting a kind of hangover from the food. When I woke up in the morning, I was bloated and sick. I was doing all this random eating, eating without thinking, just trying to make myself feel better. Now I consciously make decisions about what I put in my mouth.

Fat can also make you feel like you are in control. Ironic, isn't it? But those double stuff Oreos "make us feel so much better" as you eat them— as though you can actually control our emotions through food. You find yourself actually trying to deal with stressful situations by eating.

Hiding your "stuff"

Fat "protects" you from people—it acts like a physical barrier that actually blocks emotional intimacy. In my case, I wanted a boyfriend, but I hid— my body, my issues—behind fat. That way people wouldn't get too close to me because if they knew about all my "stuff" they wouldn't like me anyway.

I could also hide behind my job. There was my excuse to be fat. Of course. I had no time to exercise so it's okay for me to be fat right now. When I had all my belongings stolen, it was okay for me to use food to calm me down and ease my depression. I had a mother who had no time for me and still doesn't. I have nothing else—except the food.

Fat shields you from what might be the real issue or issues in your life that you just haven't faced yet.

To be fit and healthy, you have to be conscious of your food choices. You have to be aware. I will come home from traveling or from giving lectures somewhere and I'll be so exhausted in mind and body. I'll think, I feel like eating. But I stop myself and ask, are you physically hungry? If you're not, what is it that you really want? In a case where I'm tired, I usually just want to be comforted or to sleep. I drink hot tea instead, especially if it's late at night. Hot tea with lemon is very comforting to me. But I have to think about it. Otherwise, I can just sit down and eat.

Through tough practice day by day, I got to the point where I was able to ask myself, what is it I am feeling at the moment that makes me want to eat? Until you know that, until you can get to the point of asking yourself that when you feel the need to eat, you will just continue in your destructive cycle of eating and feeling miserable about yourself. My mom had a bumper sticker she kept on the wall. It said, "if hunger is not the problem, food is not the answer." And that really rings true today because I have taken the time to become conscious of my choices.

It's also about hunger management. If I have appointments from one to five in the afternoon, but it's only 11:30 and I'm not hungry, I have to think, no I'm not hungry now, but I *will* be, so I need to eat something because starving myself isn't going to get me anywhere. Now that I am home writing all the time or on the computer answering e-mails, I could eat all day. Not only is eating great for procrastination, it's also a great way to kill time. That's another way of masking what's really going on, what you're really feeling, with food.

You need to get in touch with those feelings that send you to food in the first place. When you look at yourself and you say, I feel fat, that just means that you are transferring your inability—and it may be quite natural depending on what you have gone through in your life—to deal with why you are eating to the problem only being about your physical body. That's when you fall into the trap of thinking that if you just lost weight you would be a happier, more fulfilled person.

Cultural influences
Dieting
We live in a world that does a multi-billion dollar business in dieting and diet products every year. American culture in particular pushes dieting and has ever since they found out they could make big bucks doing it. Diets are no longer just fads, they are strenuous, panicked ways of life for women

mind body spirit

as young as ten years old. We need to stop once and for all and recognize that diets:

- don't work at all;
- work for a little while and then set us up for later failure; or
- work but are an unhealthy way of achieving a lower body weight (and have nothing to do with dealing with the person we are inside).

Let's be honest with ourselves, one step at a time. Most of us have stepped inside the door of a weight control program at some point in our lives and we know, deep inside, that it's just wishful thinking. My experience with weight loss programs varied. Think about what it takes to get you to that door. For me, it was, okay, that's it; I have to do something. I would go in and feel humiliated that I couldn't do it alone. I'd feel that going through their door was admitting defeat.

I filled out the questionnaire, went to the consultations, suffered through the group therapy, listening as other people talked about their week and how hard it was to break their hand to mouth cycle.

In one case (I'd prefer not to name names), I felt like as long as I was eating this particular program's food—that included freeze dried food, powders, etc.—I was okay. Consequently, I lost weight and kept it off for about three or four months. But when I went out into the "real world" of eating, I was screwed.

In another program (that I loved when I stayed on it the right way), I ate real food. It adapted you for real life, but it was still a diet. I thought, I don't want to pay someone $20 to weigh me every week. I'm accountable to me and I don't need someone checking up on me. At least not that someone.

Just Do It mentality

Our world tries to convince us that all we need to do to lose weight is get up and exercise. From the standpoint that we create our own discipline, that yes, we do need to go from horizontal to vertical in the morning, it's a valid catch-phrase. But it doesn't address the emotional issues tied to weight. It doesn't help you come to terms with the idea of becoming conscious of your daily choices.

If I were to guess who was fat because of issues they hadn't addressed and who was just plain lazy, I would think it was about half and half. In other words, some people are out there using food as comfort and some people are just eating what they want and are not willing to get up and do the work.

Our bodies as objects

Our world encourages and capitalizes upon objectifying and exploiting the female body, preferably in waif-like form. Is it any wonder that our own self-esteem and view of our own body is so contingent upon what we see in magazines? You have choices. You don't have to buy into the magazines' consumer view of our bodies. You don't have to accept that what is on those glossy colored pages is our model of perfection. You also don't have to hate those women on those pages for being thin, because you can recognize that thin doesn't mean happy.

I have heard about the lives of models. Smoking gets them through times that they want to eat, but can't because of the constant pressure to look good—perfect, really. Others eat lettuce and drink water for lunch. In other words, they starve themselves. As young as some of these girls start, it's understandable that they would be influenced by the crazy world around them. I think it's a glamorous industry, but I don't perceive that as happiness. I couldn't stand the pressure of being judged on how I look every day.

I look at other women and I say, she has great arms, good legs, or a nice smile. I notice people's bodies and I appreciate how much work it takes to achieve a fit body. I grew up in southern California, land of the perfect people. People were always, tan, fit, in shorts. I would travel to the corporate headquarters for the company I was working for at the time and I would think, God, everyone's fat here. I think growing up in an atmosphere where I perceived that everyone around me was perfect internalized a lot of pressure for me to be that way, too. And of course, I couldn't.

Total number of overweight adults (20-74 years old): Approximately 58 million Americans (about one-third)

Percentage of adult American men trying to lose weight at any given time: 20-24 %

Percentage of adult American women trying to lose weight at any given time: 35-40 %

Amount of money spent by Americans annually on weight-reduction products and services, including diet foods, products and programs: $33 billion

NATIONAL INSTITUTE OF DIABETES AND DIGESTIVE AND KIDNEY DISEASES, A BRANCH OF THE NATIONAL INSTITUTE OF HEALTH (1999)

Role of women

Our world encourages and advocates the role of women as passive pleasers. Women are seen as "moms, wives, girlfriends, lovers, etc" all in the name of submission to another. You can demand the right to be seen as a

mind body spirit

woman and as a person with your own identity, not some extension of another person. Society expects us to do more as women, and in some ways, that's an acknowledgement that women *can* do more and are capable of unbelievable achievement. Unfortunately, this can come at the expense of your sanity and can contribute to feelings of resentment that are often expressed in eating. You can set limits on what you do for others and not be called selfish, but instead be seen as self-caring.

Reasons to stop using fat & start changing your life

Physical health

It is a fact that obesity can lead to heart disease, the number one killer of women in this country. Obesity can also lead to adult onset diabetes. These and other health risks are in most cases entirely preventable. In addition, you physically don't feel good when you are overweight—you are lethargic, tired, and maybe even depressed. I know it is really easy to ignore these words. You probably don't think anything will really happen to you, so it is easy for you to keep putting off life changes. For your own sake, for your sanity in the long run, think again!

Mental health

When you get up in the morning and look at yourself, are you beating yourself up emotionally for the way that you look? If you take baby steps, achieving real goals, no matter how small, you won't need to beat yourself up because the change will be self-evident. Instead of hiding behind "figuring out what my food issue is," you'll find that as you exercise and eat healthy, you'll be amazed at what is revealed to you. If you are eating so much that you are fat, then say to yourself, that is what I do. Now what am I going to do about it? How am I going to start making better choices? What baby steps am I going to take first? You have to start somewhere and build on what you start with.

Self-love

Above all, who is the most important person to take care of in this life? YOU. So don't be fooled that paying attention to your needs, desires, wishes, dreams, etc. is selfish. If you don't take care of you, who will? And furthermore, although you want to think like I just said, you may be sadly ingrained with the habit of not loving. Love is not attention from outside sources; love comes when you trust yourself and someone *can* help bring that out in you. Notice I said, bring that out *in* you. It is there, just waiting. It just hasn't come out yet.

Letting go of fear

Fear of just about everything. Fear of not getting approval, fear of not being liked, fear of failure, fear of risking yourself and being vulnerable, fear of having love, fear of not having love, fear of feeling guilty, fear of confrontation, fear of others' judgment upon you, fear of hurting other people's feelings, etc. You might even be afraid of what you would feel like after you lost a lot of weight! Fear is a normal and natural feeling. It is valid. What you do about your fear is what defines your level of happiness or unhappiness in this world.

Making the transition

1   The first and often hardest step to take is to admit that you have a weight problem. In other words, you have a tough time dealing with life and choose to use food to cope.

2   Next step is to decide what you want to do about it and why.

3   Next step is to make a realistic plan for yourself that isn't just about exercise, but is a whole body approach to changing your life patterns one step at a time.

4   Once ensconced in your fitness regimen, how do you deal with the changes that happen in your mind, body and soul? Changing your body, after all, is more than just a physical thing. All of a sudden, the way that you look at yourself is changed, too. The way that you perceive others look at you is changed.

Action steps toward life changes

Understand your behavior patterns

Why is it that you feel like you want to go to the pantry and unearth that hidden box of chocolate? It's not the chocolate that is "bad" and you aren't "bad," so what is it? What's making you feel like you feel and act like you do? This is a combination action and feeling step because it means you need to listen to your heart and soul. Don't let your mind constantly step in, brandishing a whip, to tell you that you are "bad" because of what you

mind   body   spirit

eat. Only by understanding your patterns can you make adjustments that are healthy for you, whether it is changing the things you eat or changing the amount you eat.

How can you start to understand your patterns? Ask yourself some questions you may not want to answer. When you are standing there in the kitchen with the bag of chips in your hand, ask yourself, how did I get here? Why am I eating this? Is it because I am hungry or am I feeling sad, lonely, depressed, angry, or something else? Then *listen* to that inner voice when it answers. This is your first step toward changing your eating patterns.

And then how is it that you can reach a point at which you can stop your behavior patterns long enough to listen to that inner voice? I hope it doesn't take a crisis in your case, but so many times when something finally happens to our health, that is the low point that we need to reach to make a change.

I wrote down everything I ate, but besides that, I wrote in my journal every night about how I was feeling and different thoughts and feelings I had had during the day. I started correlating my feelings with my desire for food. That's when I started questioning my need to eat versus my actual physical hunger. I asked what do you want? My mind would give me the answers and I would deal with that.

Set boundaries

This does not mean punishing yourself for your transgressions. It means that you set limits on the expectations you have for yourself. Are you working compulsively and subsequently ending up eating your meals from McDonalds at your desk? Are you working so late that you eat right before you go to bed, standing up at the counter? Have you made so many promises to so many people that you feel like your back is starting to cave in and the only way you can stay calm is to eat chocolate?

Give yourself time for just you. Give yourself something to look forward to, something that isn't work—and I mean, your job or your house or family work. If you set healthy boundaries for yourself, then you will naturally extend those healthy boundaries to others.

Take baby steps forward

This is what you do when you set a realistic goal for yourself, whether it is eating one or two fruits and vegetables a day or making it to two glasses of water a day. These are no minor achievements; they are your baby steps toward your bigger goal—your overall mental and physical health.

I found it helped me to get out of bed easier if the night before I had laid out all my clothes in the other room so I wouldn't have the excuse that everything was put away and I had to hunt for it. This saved me the time and the excuses I would invariably try to make.

I recommend taking one small step every day. Say that you work nine to five and at 3 o'clock, you go out to the vending machine to get a chocolate bar. Maybe you get that to power yourself through the rest of the day or maybe you get the chocolate to help with the stress from the beginning of the day. Try this small baby step. Bring a healthy snack, like an orange, an apple, or an energy bar, and eat that at 3pm instead of taking the trip to the vending machine. If that means that you purposely have to leave your loose change at home so that you won't be tempted by the vending machine's eager coin slots, and that works for you, do it! But at least have a substitute and something to look forward to.

Another small step is to drink one glass of water each day. Your body needs water anyway and an interesting thing will happen. The more water you drink, the more your body will regulate the amount of water it demands. Think of water as a purifier. If you can drink just one glass (say, eight or ten ounces) a day, then that is one more baby step toward your overall goal of health.

Say, no more excuses

Reach a point within yourself where you can say—stand in front of a mirror if you have to and look yourself right in the eye—no more excuses! Because when you realize that your world is filled with excuses, filled with reasons not to do something, even if it is in your best interest, you have taken an action step for yourself.

I got sick of being a victim. I was letting excuses stop me from getting what I wanted: a healthy, balanced life with people in it who loved me and who I loved. I was young and out of shape. I would take a cab from my hotel to the convention center when the convention center was a block away. My life was ridiculous until that fateful day when I owned my actions. I owned them and I owned *up* to them. And I stamped the words, No More Excuses permanently in my brain, so they would always be there when I felt weak.

mind body spirit

See your inner willpower

By this, I mean, "will" and "power," i.e., the will within yourself to make a change, any change, and the power that will gives you. When you direct your will in a way that is healthy for your mind body and soul, you are giving yourself a tremendous amount of power. I also believe what one of my Connectors told me and that is willpower is the willingness to work. The discipline comes from the doing; it doesn't arrive Federal Express. You have to go after it. And it won't be easy and it *will* be a daily struggle until it becomes a daily habit.

Express yourself

What are the most important things in your life? I would guess your feelings. And if you cannot or will not express those feelings and communicate them to others in a healthy and positive way, you can't feel good about yourself. This will build up your feelings of rage, resentment, self-hatred, depression, etc. and you may have the tendency to "stuff" food into yourself much like you are holding back your feelings.

The first few mornings that my alarm blared out at 5am, Martin complained and got upset. So I conveniently worked it out in my head—and this rationalization is so easy—that I just turned off the alarm and went back to sleep. But something had changed. I couldn't really put a finger on it, but those first few days when I rolled over and went back to sleep, I felt awful about myself. I spent most of the day beating myself up because I had been so determined to make my newfound program a success and here I was falling back into my old habits again. But what could I do? It wasn't fair to wake him up just because I supposedly said I was going to exercise.

So I decided to call a meeting. Yep, that's right, a meeting! I called Martin at work and asked if we could schedule a meeting to discuss some important issues. You could have heard a pin drop on the other end of the phone. I found out later he thought I was breaking up with him. We met over dinner and I told him I really wanted to give this exercise and healthy lifestyle a chance. If I was willing to get my fat butt up at 5am, the least he could do is support me in doing so and not complain about the alarm clock going off and waking him up.

This meeting went easier than I thought. Finally a boyfriend who was on my side. He just wanted me to be happy and he was so used to my half-hearted attempts at losing weight that he never knew whether to believe me or not. I would say one thing and do another. He just didn't want me to set myself up for failure again and have to be there to console me when it happened.

This time I was serious. I shocked myself with how serious and how determined I felt inside. So now I have Martin's blessing. But I wouldn't have had that and, more importantly, I wouldn't have had my own action step if I had not expressed how I felt about it in a reasonable way. I was able to air my feelings about my weight loss plans and I actually got support in return.

I know that expressing this kind of thing is a risk. As I said, there were many times that I would say I was going to do something and I didn't follow through or I gave up. Give yourself the permission to feel safe enough to express your feelings and thoughts. In doing so, you are moving forward, even if you have to say it a few times to really get started on a healthy path.

Get active

Find an activity that makes you happy and makes you move. Whether it is walking around the block, riding a bike down a nature trail, or dancing like crazy to your favorite music, this is about getting your body involved with your heart and soul. Incorporate that very human part of you— body—with that wonderful spiritual part of you—soul.

I think you'll be surprised to find that the more you do, the more you'll want to do! And you will enjoy doing it because it's something that is already a part of you. Or try an activity that you have always wondered about but have been afraid to try. Throw that fear out by thinking, there is no worst case scenario here. There is no judge and jury. There is just me doing something that I not only like, but is good for me, too.

I bought a treadmill late one night while channel surfing. I saw this infomercial featuring a treadmill that folded up to save space. What a great idea! I bought it and of course used it once or twice before it became the clothes hanger that it remains for so many of you.

I set a goal for myself. Just a small one! My goal was to walk one mile on my treadmill each morning. That took about 20 minutes. Each morning the alarm would go off at 5am and I would drag myself out of bed. I remember it being so hard to go from horizontal to vertical. That's the hardest step. After that everything seemed to flow. But I would lay in my nice warm bed trying to talk myself out of my workout. Sometimes I would win the argu-

mind   body   spirit

ment, but most of the time I lost. A few weeks went by and I got my little taste of success. One mile became easy. I even started venturing outside every so often because the treadmill got boring.

It doesn't matter whether you have to watch television or wear a Walkman as you walk on a treadmill, as long as you are doing something.

Grocery items

The basic rule is that if you don't buy the food and it's not in your house, it makes it really easy *not* to eat it. I don't know how many times I bought groceries and items I knew darn well would call my name from the pantry shelves. I would eat whatever the items were, then beat myself up over not having willpower. Do yourself a favor and don't buy the chips, chocolate bars, frozen pizza, and ice cream in the first place. If it's not in the house, you're not eating it, and you're not punishing yourself mentally for it.

If you did buy it, fish around in those dark corners and closets and throw it out! Go down the street to a trash can outside of a bank or grocery store if you're afraid you might fish around in your own trash to retrieve what you got rid of.

Instead fill your house with healthy foods. Plenty of fruits and vegetables is always a great place to start. If you're hungry enough, you'll eat them. Funny thing, your body will actually begin to crave those healthy food items, instead of the junk you've been throwing it and calling that food.

Scheduling

How do you fit exercise into your already filled-to-the-top jar of priorities? The answer for me is early morning. Now before you slam the book shut and throw it across the room, remember I didn't start out with morning exercise either, but if I had it to do over again, I would start with morning exercise from the get go. When you work out first thing in the morning, it's over and done with. That sets your day. Nothing else can come up to move your exercise off your to-do list. If you have children and you schedule your exercise first thing in the morning, you won't have to worry about any surprises that come up during the day.

On a physical level, morning exercise rules. Getting your metabolism revved from the beginning can really do wonders for you the rest of the day. And don't worry if you don't start out being a morning exerciser. Just moving at all is a triumph and you can always fine tune goals and habits as you progress along.

My biggest motivation is knowing that it is realistically then or never. The odds that I will find time later in the day are slim and none. I have gotten to the point that when I can't get out of bed, I make myself acknowledge that I have made a conscious choice not to exercise that day; I don't let myself slip into rationalizing that I will do it later, etc. Sometimes just putting that much thought into the decision not to get up wakes me up enough to go ahead and get up.

ELIZABETH, CONNECTING IN NC

Time is the one area where we are all equal. Regardless of your age, weight, religion, or social status, we all have 24 hours in a day and seven days in a week. It's one area where we're all on a level playing field. Now sure we all have different things that fill our days, but we can choose what those things are.

If you can't muster the strength to exercise in the morning, how about lunchtime? You see women in skirts and tops with Reeboks on their feet, power walking during the noon hour, and you know that they're fitting their exercise in, come what may. Any 20 to 30 minutes you can find just for you will reap many rewards. Once you get a small taste of how great you feel when you do it consistently, you'll want more.

When I first started, I would come home from work and walk on the treadmill at something like two mph, watching television while I was doing it. That helped time go by more quickly. I only did it for about 20 minutes at first, then I was off and ready for dinner. I kept this routine going for a few weeks, only getting off track if I had to work late or had an out of town business trip. So I did the best I could.

When I finally made a decision to work out in the mornings, I found I was going to bed earlier to make it easier to get up in the morning. A small, subtle change. Once I was working out in the morning, I was making better food choices throughout the day and there was no longer a nagging thought like "I should work out today" in my head. And the discipline you acquire making this happen extends to other areas of your life as well.

mind body spirit

CHAPTER 3

Living the commitment

I wore shorts out in public for the first time in many years today! Unfortunately my legs were rubbing together so badly I developed a horrible rash, but I think it's a HUGE step that I was out in public wearing shorts! I'm still very apprehensive about showing up at different events. I don't feel like I belong yet. But the more I show up and participate, the more pride I feel. I feel I must lead by example and give others hope that they belong out at events wearing shorts also. I'd love to change the perception of what an athlete looks like.

I'm feeling very good about myself lately. I'm making really good choices everyday and my insides are finally catching up with my outsides. Yet, I still get "the look" when I talk about working out around various people. That hurts. I know they don't believe me when I tell them I'm trying to start a running program. So, I do it quietly and silently and one day I'll show em! But, for now, it's not important what OTHERS think of me, it's more important of what I THINK OF ME! Such a huge step on this journey!

JOURNAL ENTRY, AUGUST 29, 1997

I pulled my car into a space in a parking lot littered with teenagers, standing in after-school groups, swigging coffee or ice lattes. I'm sure my mind was a million miles away, what with all the pressures of work and keeping up my daily exercise routine. I felt the cool rush of air conditioning as I opened the door into Starbucks. The line wasn't too long and I got into it willingly. Behind me, more gaggles of teenagers, dressed in baggy pants, torn jeans and t-shirts laughed and talked loudly.

Suddenly, as I was standing there minding my own business, I heard the words, "if she's going to wear a shirt like that, she should at least be fit!" The group then burst into peals of laughter. Well, they were referring to me. I was wearing jeans and a t-shirt that said, "a fit woman is a powerful woman" on the front.

The first thing I felt was humiliation and shame. Of course I shouldn't have been wearing such a brash statement when I still had a roll of fat around my belly and a big butt. My mind tried telling me this first. After all, I still had a ways to go, even if I had come a long ways already. I still had such a long way to go, despite the 100 pounds I had already shed, despite

mind 🏃 body 🏃 spirit 🏃

the fact that I fought for and had the discipline to get up and exercise every morning at 5am, despite the fact that I was slowly becoming someone I could like. Never mind all that. Obviously, the people around me still saw me as just one thing: fat.

I felt like the whole café was staring at me. So I decided to make the most of the opportunity.

Turning around, I walked up to the table, around which were seated three or four lithe, young girls, none of whom could have been older than 15 or 16. I saw one look down into her coffee as I approached, nervously stirring it with a straw, avoiding my eyes.

"Pardon me, but I heard what you said. I just finished my second marathon. And any time that you would like to run 20 miles, give me a call." I said this loud enough for the whole place to hear, and then flourished one of my Connectors business cards.

The rest of the people in Starbucks cheered and the girls were red-faced and silent.

Don't get me wrong. I didn't set out to be malicious or to seek revenge. I guess what happened is that it became a flag post for every other time that someone had looked through me on the street, had whispered how fat I was as I walked by, had judged me by the way I looked and decided I wasn't their type of person. I finally hit the wall.

Here I was, in my early thirties, finally getting my act together—physically, mentally and spiritually—and now this. Boy did I see clearly just how people had been viewing me all my life. This was my opportunity to tell them, guess what, I'm *not* that person. You don't know me at all. You don't know who I am and you don't know where I came from to get where I am now.

We have *all* been there. In fact, there's no guarantee that we won't be there again at some point during our journey toward health and fitness. Once you make the decision, you might even be okay for a while. Then something in your life will interfere—and life brings along a lot to interfere with our commitment to ourselves. How do you make sure that you are living your commitment once you have made it? What can get you going and keep the fire burning under you? I will share some of what has worked for me and for others, especially Connectors.

Getting going

In the beginning, I was motivated to lose weight. That's what kept me going, avoiding the 300-pound mark on the scale. But that wasn't enough. I had lost weight before and it hadn't been enough, and worse, I hadn't kept it off. I was blind to my path, my method, my plan of action. If you can't see the way, how can the way see you? Everyone can fantasize what it is like to reach a successful destination. The reality is, can you see the path that leads you there?

Baby steps, consistent baby steps—that is the path that leads to the goals you fantasize about. It's the getting up when you don't feel like it. It's the little more 'push' when you don't think you have anything left.

How often do we make up our mind about something before we even give it a fighting chance? A big part of keeping your commitment to yourself is living in the moment, experiencing joy every day. How can we do that if we're crossing bridges before we come up to them? It's a tough struggle for us as humans because we have this tendency I think to want to control everything. Instead, just take one day at a time, even one hour at a time if you have to. Say to yourself, I will deal with that when it happens—or *if* it happens—but until then I will not worry or be anxious over it.

Adjusting your mindset like this will make you breathe a little easier. If you give yourself permission to take one day at a time, you will find that you get to your goals much faster. And you open yourself up to the possibilities, not the limitations.

Say that you want to try something, like golf or tennis, and you want to take the time for yourself, to take lessons. You are worth that effort—what is the worst thing that can happen? Ask yourself what you would be doing if you knew you could not fail? And what is the worst thing that could happen? You would be out the money and the time for the lessons. Big deal! You'll never know what you can do until you *do it!*

The same goes for your fitness and health program. Just take that first baby step. Just give yourself the right to take care of *you*.

Inspiration

I think many of you are like me, and we read something and "get inspired" but after a few weeks, well, ya know, "things" get in the way, *otherwise known as excuses!*

mind body spirit

No matter how successful I am, I always will have a problem staying motivated, because I hate exercise and love to eat. Recently I had another true test of my motivation. For some reason, I did NOT want to go out and exercise. I wasn't making excuses; I just didn't want to do it...too lazy, I guess. I knew that if I were going to get myself out of this mode, I would need to consult my fellow Florida Connectors. I went online and...I just poured out my heart. Yes, this was difficult and left me vulnerable, because I told them that I had time, I had the place, and the ideal situation to exercise, but I just didn't want to do it. I asked for suggestions on how to do some "self talk" to get the motivation to go out and walk. So many Connectors responded to me with such words of encouragement that I couldn't help but "catch the fever." By the end of the week I had gotten out the door and...I even signed up to walk the half marathon at Disney World.   PATRICIA, CONNECTING IN FL

So, what do I do?

I like the part of me that gets inspired by watching a movie or reading a good book, so that's good! It allows me to think of what is possible. I celebrate that part of me. What I do is set a small goal. If I decide that I really am inspired to do "x" (whatever "x" is), I don't try to do it all in one week. I learned the hard way that it doesn't work that way.

The other "secret" for me is and I don't know how many different ways I can say this, over and over and over again: *check in daily.* Accountability is key! Select somebody and work together to hold each other accountable. Use your local Connectors to check in. Some Connectors call each other daily and check in. Some check in via e-mail. Whatever works.

Post your goals each week and check in daily. I set small, baby step goals to get me to where I want to go. Then I check in daily. Why? Because *life* is daily. It's that basic. The daily choices you make will get you to the goal you say you want.

That inspiration you found once or twice will come and go. Feelings are fluid. Don't wait till you "feel like it." Trust me; that won't happen very often, if you're like me. I schedule workouts for my really long runs with other people. I know I'll show up if I have to meet others, plus it's just more fun and we go out to eat afterwards!

It's a great thing to be inspired, but I want to hear what the Connectors are doing with the inspiration. Then, when we read something that inspires us, we join in! We know we can do it, too and we want to know how and we want people to experience the joy of accomplishing something with us and cheer for us every step of the way.

It's thrilling to read about someone's inspiring story. Now take it up a notch and go live that inspiration!

What's the deal with these Connectors?

In her book, *Make the Connection,* Oprah presents steps for losing weight and improving your life. As a group, the Connectors are committed to "making the connection" together, that is, following the advice in Oprah's book and helping each other to make better lives. We have men and women of all ages, shapes, sizes, religions and fitness levels. All are welcome because everyone has to start somewhere.

It's easy to join the Connectors. Read *Make the Connection,* sign up for the email thought for the day, subscribe to a Connector's e-mail discussion group in your region, or use the Connector's message boards for discussion and support. My thought for the day, which at current count goes out to close to 20,000 Connectors — whew! — is a piece of inspiration, motivation, humor or true experience from me (and other sources) that is designed to give you a daily boost of support in your fitness journey and life.

The Connectors' impact

Average people let the obstacles stop them from going after what they want. They listen to the doubters. They let their jobs rule their lives. I am surrounded by all of the Connectors who refuse to settle for less! They truly are the "wind beneath my wings." They are my purpose and my reason for continuing on. I lead by example, so when I don't want to do something, I think, "I don't want to let the Connectors down." And I do it.

I want to hear what the Connectors are doing with the inspiration because it inspires me. That's why I love to get the brag reports at the end of each month. What sets the Connectors apart from any other "weight loss group" is the Connector spirit.

And, secondly, the Connectors themselves lead by example. We don't profess to have all the answers, but we're here to lead the way and we hold the door open for others to come join us.

The importance of a support group

It's cheering and supporting others as they struggle to reach their goals that makes reaching your goals all the sweeter! I'm here cheering for each

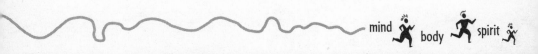
mind body spirit

and every one of you every step of the way, whether you're a Connector or not. And who doesn't need cheerleaders?

I think it's a valuable thing to know you can log on any time, day or night and write to others who are out in the trenches with you every step of the way. They are cheering for your every success and holding out a hand for you to grasp when you fall down and scrape your knee.

No, we're not perfect—far from it—but we are here to support and offer advice and encouragement. All you have to do is show up and do your part and offer support and encouragement too. To me, the Connectors are people like me who are trying to be healthy and make choices on a daily basis. To have their support is like having someone hold a hand out, grab my hand, and say, okay, Tawni, you can do it, let's keep going, let's keep going *together*.

HOPE

I am full of hope now, but it wasn't always that way. I felt hopeless most of the time. Because of my high expectations, of others and of myself, I sensed that I was a failure a majority of the time. I was always comparing myself to my mom and I would never measure up. The minute I would try to get ahead, the car would break down, a large tax bill would come, or some other hurdle that I would feel totally overwhelmed by. It got to the point where I was sure that if I looked up, there would be a little black cloud right above my head; that's how cursed I thought I was.

> "The very least you can do in your life is to figure out what you hope for. And the most you can do is live inside that hope. Not admire it from a distance, but live right in it, under its roof."
>
> BARBARA KINGSOLVER

My attitude turned around and the way I approached life changed. One of the psychologists that I went to gave me some homework one time that has stayed with me. He said, Tawni, just get up in the morning and brush your teeth. If you can do that, you get a gold star for the day; you get to put that on your calendar. When I was able to bring in a calendar filled with shiny foil stars, I knew that I was on the road to recovering my hope.

The key is to take it on a minute level. Don't try to do it all at once; just do what you think you can do, no matter how small. For me it made me think differently about achieving anything. I got up, showered, dressed, worked, and ate. If I went for a walk, even to the end of the block and back, that was a small success.

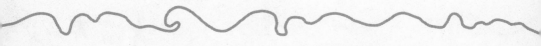

I started seeing I was successful and that gave me hope. After that I started to set goals. That led to more success and—you guessed it—more goals. It was a positive, powerful domino effect in which the dominoes falling were like building blocks for my confidence.

We are so mean to ourselves every day. "Why the hell bother?" "It doesn't matter because I didn't lose any weight." "I should have run today, but I didn't." Turning this around with small goals and small successes leads to a joyful spirit. I got rid of that chip on my shoulder, was filled with positive energy, and began inspiring other people instead of hiding out and concentrating my focus on everything that was wrong with the world and with my life.

I hope to be a life-changing influence because it is my way of giving back. When we feel better about ourselves, when we hold hope in our hearts, we are better wives, better husbands, and better employees. It acts like a ripple effect through our whole life.

Motivation is a welcome wind at your back. But winds are changeable and fickle; motivation comes and goes. Will is a faithful friend, at your side in both the sunlit days and dark nights of the soul, speaking quietly of what is important and good. You can depend upon your will because it comes from within you.

So sail the winds of motivation when they blow, but in the calms and dry spells, rely on your will to carry you through.

DAN MILLMAN, AUTHOR OF EVERYDAY ENLIGHTENMENT

COURAGE

I have a wonderful pneumonic for courage I have listed below. Besides what I have listed, courage means asking for what you want and going after what you want. It means standing up for yourself.

To make a decision takes courage. To get up at 5am before work to exercise is a decision you have to make every day, so decisions are a *huge* step in all of this.

I had to banish the word "failure" from my vocabulary because I don't believe in failure—only results! If I can change what I do, I can always get a different result. Some of the greatest miracles of my life have not come about by grand events, but rather by the little things I have chosen to do on a daily basis. And let me tell you, that takes courage! I know it took courage for you to decide to make a change in your life. All these fears and insecurities probably went through your head and maybe you thought you weren't brave enough, or that you didn't have it in you to make a change. But you

mind body spirit

do. You had the courage to move off the track you were on and you're here reading this, so give yourself credit. You're braver than you think.

I believe it also takes courage to *try again* when things haven't worked out the way you think they should. When I had given up after the U-Haul incident, I thought, what's the point, I always gain the weight back anyway, so why bother? Recommitting to a goal that you think is important to you is a courageous act.

Voicing your decision and your commitment to others can be daunting. You are looking for their support and encouragement, but at the same time, you might be afraid of their rejection of your idea. Continuing in the face of "nay sayers" is a huge act of courage and bravery.

Most of us just want the "quick fix." I know I did. We don't want to hear how much hard work is involved. Well, guess what? It's hard work! It takes courage every day to get up and keep going! It is easier to eat whatever you want and sleep in. Simple. Does that bring you joy? Are you happy settling for that? How does it feel to be out of breath when you play with your kids or walk up a flight of stairs? The courage to keep going on a daily basis—that is what you strive for. Think of this: you are getting out of bed and exercising, you are eating healthy and that is more than at least one other person in the world is doing. And that takes courage to step away from the norm and go after what you need for yourself!

C is for confronting people or situation

O is for overcoming obstacles

U is for understanding risks

R is for risk taking

A is for always believing in yourself

G is for goal-setting & going the distance

E is for expecting the best

Staying motivated

I'm asked over and over again, "What makes you so different than anybody else in regards to losing weight?"

I say nothing, except I don't give up. I take my frustrations and I just keep going. Every time I gave up in the past I ended up sinking lower and lower, and even in my worst of frustrations, it's not as bad as my low times when I gave up on my life.

Always good to put things in perspective. And I don't know about any of you, but often times I make things harder than they have to be. I'm learning after years of trials and tribulations, to just flow with it. I know I'm going to get frustrated, so what, who cares, it really is a part of the journey.

The "trick" is not to give up when you're frustrated the most. Those that quit almost always will come back and say they wish they had stuck with it. So, why not just stick with it?

Excuses are the easy part

I love the excuse, well, after the holidays I'll get back on track. Or, I've been so busy with work on this or that project that I haven't been able to work out. These kinds of excuses fall into the realm of "life is daily." What does that mean? I think of it in terms of brushing your teeth. Do you stop brushing your teeth because it's the holiday season? Do you stop brushing your teeth when you go on vacation? Get a job promotion? Have a death in the family?

"Life shrinks or expands in proportion to our courage."

ANAIS NIN

"The miracle isn't that I finished. The miracle is that I had the courage to start."

JOHN "THE PENGUIN" BINGHAM

Whenever I find myself thinking I'm too busy or something else (life) gets in my way, I remind myself that I always brush my teeth. No matter how tired I am, I always brush my teeth because that to me is just part of my routine. I wouldn't feel right if I *didn't* do it. Just like exercise. I know that if I *do* skip a day, I just feel weird, like something is missing.

Never give up, but give in

We all are going to have days when we don't feel like pushing ourselves to the next level and that's okay. Each day push yourself at whatever level you can for that day. And then strive to improve on the day before and build on your baby steps.

When I first started changing my patterns, I used to drink a six-pack of Diet Pepsi everyday. Well, I knew that if I was going to be working out consistently, my body needed water. I hated drinking water. Ick. So, I started with committing to drinking five Diet Pepsis and then I'd drink one glass of water, then the next week, I'd only drink four Diet Pepsis etc. And pretty soon I wasn't drinking any Pepsi and I was drinking water. Baby steps.

Just drag that body out of bed and the mind will follow. I go kicking and screaming most mornings, but I *never* have regretted it after I'm done. A little trick I use when I have a really bad case of the "I don't wannas" is to tell myself, I'll just go for a slow walk around the block to wake up, clear my mind and get the juices flowing. As I'm getting dressed, I'm still whining, so I keep repeating my small mental booster. Heck, we *all* need a mental boost from time to time!

mind body spirit

Don't try to do everything all at once. That sets you up for failure. Thinking in "black and white" can be very dangerous. Life is grey. Remember there is no finish line; there is only the continuing path, winding though it may be. This is about developing healthy habits for life. This is about creating the best life possible for each of you. Making your health a priority will spill over to other areas in your life. Trust me on that!

Nurturing yourself & others

When you get up in the morning, face that mirror. It's okay; we're going to change it from your enemy to your friend. This is your way of seeing yourself and I challenge you to throw out that resident voice that beats you up emotionally for how you look. Evict that thing! There's no room for it here anymore. Instead, take a look. Everyone has at least one good thing about themselves. Whether this is a physical or a mental positive, I encourage you to say it when you look in the mirror.

For instance, if you look at yourself, you can say, I really have pretty hair. My arms are really looking good from that weightlifting. If you just got a manicure, maybe your toes look fantastic. There's *always* something! Or in your head. God, I did a great job on that project at work. I really keep my house orderly. I'm really good at sewing. Praise yourself. You need this; it's not selfish, it's self-caring.

I like to give back to myself, to nurture myself, and it's a reward really. When I exercise, that is for me. When I am doing my stretching and warming up before a run, I think about my day and what it will hold. I think about the Connectors and what they are doing all over the country. This is really my alone time, just for me.

And after a run, as I am cooling down, I take time to reflect, to be quiet with my thoughts and with myself. When I was working, I rushed all the time. I rushed from bed, to exercise, to work, to bed again. Now I don't have to do that. I have the time to be meditative. But even if I had a job to go to, I would still insist on carving that time out of the day for me.

Every day I do something for someone else, whether it is a card or a phone call. I check in on someone who may be struggling because I feel so good when I give back to someone else. That is part of the reason I began the Connectors Angel Network (CAN). If someone were running his or her first 5k race, I would send a card signed "Connector Angel." Or I would send flowers or balloons. I like the idea of anonymous acts of giving on a daily basis. What is even more wonderful is that now others are doing it, too, and I feel proud that I have set something so positive in motion.

Connectors' Angel Network

I started the Connector Angel Network (CAN) in 1997 shortly after Oprah launched her Angel Network on her television show. It's a way that the Connectors can send things anonymously to support other Connectors. We send cards of congratulations, support and encouragement. We send candles, flowers, running related items (health bars, socks) and other stuff like that. Just anonymous gifts to let other Connectors know we're thinking about them. It exists for support and it's very cool to get a card or a gift in the mail knowing that somebody else is thinking about you. I just started asking Connectors to send me their mailing address if they wanted to be a part of the Connector Angel Network. I keep the master list, and that way it's safe.

When somebody wants to send somebody something they have to ask me for the address. Now that I have state leaders in every state, each leader keeps track of their own list in their area. Saves me time! I received a Connector Angel Anonymous gift of an airline ticket and hotel accommodation for my recent trip to Disney World! *Hard to believe.* I've also given airline tickets as anonymous gifts too! Starting CAN is probably one of the *best* things I've ever done.

Time for you

Although so much of my joy comes from doing things for others, there are definitely things that I like to do for myself. I take a long, relaxing bath once a week, where I light candles and listen to light jazz. I get full body massages as often as I can; nothing like that to treat yourself tenderly! I also like to get facials, manicures and pedicures because I enjoy the feeling of taking care of myself. A secret I can share with you is that if you don't have the funds to go to a beauty salon, try calling a local beauty college. I went to one and got a pedicure for only five dollars.

I have an ongoing wish list and I cross things off as I get them. Things on the list might be extra candles, a new CD, dinner at a new restaurant I am interested in, a walk in the park with Martin, etc. I believe in getting little treats and my wish list gives me something to look forward to.

I read all kinds of books, but especially motivational and inspirational books. I love the idea of taking that time for me, even if it is only 15 minutes sandwiched in here or there for a few pages of uplifting words.

mind body spirit

When I first started getting serious about making a change in my lifestyle, I used to pay myself to exercise. Each time I worked out, I put one dollar in a jar. As time, went on, I gave myself a raise and started putting ten dollars in the jar. And I didn't always put in cash. Sometimes I would write myself a check or even put down the date, what I did, and mark ten dollars on a scrap of paper and that would go in the jar. Eventually I would take the money and buy whatever I wanted with it, like a new running shirt, etc.

One of the most important things I do that is very nurturing is to block out periods of time to spend with people who are important to me. Now I know that sounds a little silly, but it has really kept my relationships in balance. I am such a whirlwind of activity that I literally have to schedule time to spend with Martin and with friends. For instance, if Martin and I have issues to discuss, we have a set time and we sit down, don't accept phone calls during that time, and can talk about what is on our minds in a calm and neutral atmosphere. That is what works for me. It's okay to set boundaries. You will be amazed at the power you feel when you do something that is healthy not only for you, but for the people around you.

Keeping a journal

Like many people, I kept a diary as a child. But that act of writing my thoughts and feelings down never became an integral part of myself until about six years ago. My journaling is a combination of a gratitude list and a flow of thoughts onto the page, a recollection of my progress day by day. My journal is a safe, non-judgmental place to express myself.

I think that no matter how busy you get, living your chaotic lives, no matter how many distractions there are, writing in a journal can be freeing, liberating. I look forward to writing in my journal and making my gratitude list no matter how tired I am. And if you have kids, you could make it into an arts and crafts project. They could create their own scrapbooks or paste together interesting shapes or words, while Mom gets her 15 minutes with her journal. I write in many different types of journals—spiral bound, plain notebooks, whatever. You might even design your own!

I write five things on my gratitude list each night before I go to bed and then I read them the next morning. These are things that I am thankful for, for instance, I am thankful for Martin, I am happy it wasn't hot when I ran, I got some really nice e-mails, etc. It can be something as simple as I am happy I got to eat Dannon lemon yogurt today.

By writing, I find that I always look for the good things. I think that changes the way I live, too, because I think, what will I write that I am thankful for tonight? That giving thanks is like being rewarded. It's wonderful to make yourself a priority in this way. You will have so much more to give to your family and friends when you give first to yourself.

Going within

I have my own form of meditation. In the morning, after the initial bleary-eyed stumbling around, after I push back the wall of resistance and rationalizations once again, I pad through the house, lighting candles. Before long, the whole house is lit with a soft glow and filled with wonderful smells. That really grounds me. As I am stretching before a run, I go over my gratitude list that I made the night before. I think about how many reasons I have for being thankful. I am thankful to God for another day in my progress toward a healthy mind and body. I take a deep breath of sweet smelling air and acknowledge the things and people that are good in my life.

Running connects me to God and to nature because as I run along, I am in awe of what is around me. In fact, it was while I was running that I had one of the most spiritual experiences of my life. I was in Big Sur, CA during the marathon, and they had a part of the race where you could run the last 10 miles of the marathon course. So there I was, doing my walk/run on an overcast day, typical of the area. As I crested the hill at mile 23, I heard the sounds of classical music (they had a gathering of players on the cliff) and their voices filled the air with singing. As I ran up the hill, it sounded like a choir of angels and I got chills. I felt like I was in heaven and I said to myself, "I am so glad to be alive."

My spirituality is about positive energy and good karma. I do read the Bible and I pray daily. I have a prayer list. I pray for courage, wisdom, strength, the right decisions, and patience (I really struggle with that one!). I pray for Martin and for his health. I also pray for certain Connectors that are going through tough times. I pray for them to understand and to have comfort, to see and learn from the experience. I pray that they come out better, not bitter.

I'm not into psychics or card reading, although I know that that can be useful for a lot of people. I have a few people that I really trust and in times of need, I call them. In terms of being with myself, I write in my journal every night and for me that is truly going within.

mind body spirit

For me, God is a higher power, outside of me, but also inside of me. I have my own relationship with God in that I believe in a power greater than myself. I try to live on a spiritual path and I believe there is a plan and a divine purpose and that everything happens for a reason.

Mental flowers

I like the idea of having something to tell yourself during those times when you "would just rather not!" I call them mental flowers. It's like getting a shot of energy and "go power" in your veins. These are the things that you tell yourself or the little things you do to keep going. And they're flowers because it's like giving yourself a gift. To be able to grab hold of a flower and say, let's go, there's no limits on what I can do, is so powerful and so beautiful.

There are plenty of days the inner child in me whines and stamps her foot and yells "I don't wanna!" but then I remind myself it really is not about "wanting," it's about "doing." If I get up in the morning (anywhere between 4:40 and 5:40 am depending on my schedule), and physically sit up in bed, take a deep breath and say "ok, let's go," I will do it. The workouts help me wake up and I think I am even more alert at work! I now sleep very well.   ALICIA, CONNECTING IN TX

It doesn't matter if I feel like exercising, because 90 percent of the time, I *don't*. But when I get up in the morning, I say to myself, "this is who I am, this is what I do." I also think of myself as an athlete in training, and for me, that is really a switch being flipped, because it takes the focus off of being overweight. I'm training for life. This builds on my success, not failure. Think about it. There is always some sort of progress, no matter how small. Six months ago, I only ran one mile; now I can run two.

I also remind myself that I am committed to my health, that my health is the number one priority in my life. Without it, I have nothing, I do nothing, I want nothing. You have probably noticed that if you don't feel good, for whatever reason, whether it is a toothache or a general fatigue, you don't care about anything else. The sole focus is on not feeling good. To make a wholehearted commitment to health makes me proud and makes sense for all areas of my life.

Goals

Set a goal. This sounds like it's overused, but it's true. Set a goal, no matter how small. Goals are your map to get you to where you're going. I didn't start out having a goal to create this wonderful group of Connectors. I selfishly went online to find a support group and I couldn't find one, so I created my own. My goal was to help myself and by leading, I was helping myself, because I thought if I was leading, I better have my act together. Somehow it gave me comfort to know that there were other people out there struggling to get their butts out of bed in the early morning, too.

Write your goals down. If you want, call it a Wish List instead of a list of goals. What do you wish? When you think of something, write it down. If you have a bad habit you want to break, you could write that down. How will you go about working on breaking that bad habit?

I write things down that I know won't get done *unless* I write them down. Once I write my wishes down, I keep them posted where I can see them every day. Each week I check in and see where I am on my goals and that way an entire month doesn't slip by with me being off track.

Focus on one small goal at a time. If you choose that your first baby step is to commit to one day of exercise a week, then that's great! Now I know what you're thinking: one day? Why bother? That won't do me any good. Don't fall into this all or nothing mentality. One day of reaching your goal has a monumental effect on your whole outlook on life.

I tend to think big, so I break down each of the big goals into smaller ones. For example, say that I want to run a 5k without stopping. I begin with walking one mile without stopping. Each week, I add half a mile to my walking routine. When I reached the point where I could comfortably walk 3-1/2 miles, I would go on the same route and jog for thirty seconds and walk for two minutes. Jog for thirty seconds and walk for two minutes. Little by little, but darn it, I did it!

BIG GOAL: Walk one mile

Baby Step Goal: Get up before work and walk for 10 minutes

How to Get There: Lay out exercise clothes the night before.

So start with that small goal and build from there. I have found that whenever I achieve these small successes my brain wants to experience more of them. Most of us squash these tiny victories as "not good enough." We beat ourselves up that we couldn't run a marathon after two weeks of starting to run. This is a journey. There is no finish line. I continue to set goals each month and I am constantly challenging myself. There's always room for improvement, but if I never started with one day, I would never have reached the starting line of my first marathon in Honolulu, HI in December 1997.

mind body spirit

Keep in mind of course, that my goals or wishes won't help you decide what *your* goals or wishes need to be. Goals are individual and need to be important to you and you alone. No comparing and no judging!

Beating the ya-buts

Once we determine what we want (the goal/dream/wish), what tends to happen is the "ya-buts" start popping up in our mind. I remember hearing Bob Greene talk about this, too. Ya but: I don't have the energy, I don't have the clothes, I don't have the time, I don't have the support around me, I'm too short, I'm too old, etc. What we need to do is turn our ya-but into a "get off your butt" activity.

Start by writing down the "ya-buts" and then move to the vision: what it would look like if it were fixed, changed or improved? Write in the positive sense. The vision or goal has to have emotion words attached to it because that is what moves us forward as humans.

The next step would be to write down the vision or goal and add, in bullet or number format, words that describe what it would look and feel like once it is completed.

For example, if your current reality is "out of shape," how does your current reality feel or look? Sluggish, lethargic, embarrassed, fat, sloppy, panting, etc. What's the goal? "In shape." What does that feel like? High energy, enthused, proud, confident, firm, toned, fit, etc. Turn that into an affirmation: I feel proud, confident, happy and energized because I exercise each and every day. I put my affirmations on bright neon index cards, read at least one every day (three, four and five times a day), visualize what that looks like, and then go and act like it.

Consistency

Do what you say you're going to do. This is how you become confident in yourself and build self-esteem. When you follow through on your plan of action, no matter how small or how grandiose, you hear this voice inside you say, you're great! See how much you can do?! One promise kept to yourself at a time. Then commit to two days a week. And then three. This is reality. Take one day at a time and do the best you can with it.

I had to ease myself into this new lifestyle gently. Remember, "power is strength over time." We're in this for a lifetime, so start from zero and you'll be amazed what you can build. Think of a newborn baby learning how to walk. Aren't we thrilled to see them take their first step? We can celebrate the same thing in ourselves as we practice consistency in exercise and health, one day at a time.

Success

Success is evolving. I have success every single day of my life: small successes. For a long time, I had this outmoded idea of success. I thought it meant climbing the corporate ladder, getting a promotion, making more money, buying things, clothes, shoes, etc. Now it means being the best person I can be. Success is in the journey. There are still qualities about myself that I work on. You can feel the glow of success when you reflect on the way your journey has been. So give yourself something to smile about. Live your success in baby steps every day.

Success is making a difference and thinking, I finally matter now. For me, it's seeing people transform their lives and hearing that it was because of something they read about me or about the Connectors. It's setting a goal and reaching it. I feel most successful when I set goals—and even if I *don't* reach the goal, the journey makes me feel successful. At least I tried. I set a goal to run a marathon in six hours. I don't even know where I came up with this idea; I just got it into my head one day before the race that it had to be six hours. Well, I finished in seven and I gave myself the mental beating of a lifetime. How could I have not finished in six hours? What was wrong with me? I was so disappointed. I had a temper tantrum and was generally cranky and depressed for a few hours following the race.

Then I thought, wait a minute. A year ago, I was in a wheelchair. A year ago, I didn't know if I would ever walk normally again, much less run. Had I never set the goal of finishing the marathon, I wouldn't even have been there. Total mental turnaround!

Since big success doesn't come overnight, you need little successes along the way. Rephrase everything in your head, the way I did that day. Change the vocabulary and the way you talk to yourself. Think of every healthy choice that you make as bringing you closer to your goal(s). Ask yourself, does this choice bring me closer or move me farther away from my ultimate goal or goals? Is eating this chocolate bar moving me closer to my ultimate goal or farther away? Is getting up to run at 5am closer or farther away? You can see that if you don't have a goal, it's easy to let yourself make bad choices.

mind body spirit

Remember what happened at Starbucks? On April 9, 1999, I got an e-mail that reminded me of my focus:

Dear Tawni,

I've wanted to write this letter to you for months but never could find enough courage to sit down and write you. Finally this afternoon when my mom came back from her first run of 1 mile and was beaming with pride, I decided I couldn't let another day go by without writing you an apology.

You see, I was one of the four teenagers in Starbucks that made fun of you a few months ago. I had no idea what a small world this world would turn out to be.

I don't ever read Runner's World *Magazine (I don't run; why would I?). Evidently, a friend of a friend of a friend of my mom's passed along the story about you and the Connectors in the February issue of* Runner's World *and on Super Bowl Sunday my mom started taking walks around the block.*

Then, for no reason my mom started getting up before we would get up to get ready for school and take her walks early in the morning. To the family's surprise she keeps getting up before we get up to get her morning exercise. The entire family has noticed a big change in our mom.

Here's where you come in. My mom never mentioned when she started taking walks around the block, WHY she was doing it. I just assumed she was "starting another diet." Just recently over dinner she was reading the article in Runner's *World. And I sat there stunned when she read the part about the teenagers making fun of "Tawni" in Starbucks because of the T-shirt she was wearing.*

I thought, "no way, it couldn't be." And when I read you were from the San Francisco/Bay Area I knew it MUST be the same person and then I felt awful. How could I have been so cruel? How could I tell my mom? Well, I didn't have to say anything; my tears gave me away. My mom asked me what was wrong and I just ran to my room. Eventually I told her about the day me and my friends were in Starbucks and you walked in with that T-shirt that says "A fit woman is a powerful woman" And we were laughing at you. I couldn't believe how confident and polite you were to us that day. We certainly didn't deserve your politeness.

I don't know when my mom has ever been more disappointed in me. I know she's raised me better than the way I acted.

Because of you and the story in Runner's World *Magazine my mom can now run 1 mile without stopping. She is very excited about an upcoming 5K race and we as a family couldn't be more proud.*

I know saying I'm sorry isn't good enough but I truly am. I had no right to try and humiliate you in public. I am deeply ashamed of my actions. Because of you and your example I am a different person today. I will no longer tolerate my friends or anybody for that matter making fun of other people regardless of the circumstances. I don't have to participate in that kind of behavior.

Thank you for being the woman that you are and helping my mom become a better and healthier mom.

CHAPTER 4
Fitness kick-start

I'm doing it! I'm waking up at 5am and walking on the treadmill before work! I can't believe I'm actually doing it! I'm dragging my butt the rest of the day but I'm getting in 5 workouts a week now! Yippppeee! I'm so darn proud of myself! I know it will become easier, but right now it's very hard exercising in the morning before work. But, I was struggling to get my workouts done after a long day and "something was always coming up." So, I feel really proud that I set a goal for November to get up before work and get my walks in. I'm walking for 20-30 minutes now! I can hardly believe it! Who knows what I'll be able to do next month? I need to venture outside and see if I can make it down the hill and back up again! Something to shoot for!

JOURNAL ENTRY, NOVEMBER 13, 1996

Armed only with gloves, a puffy down jacket and my Mickey Mouse hat, I stepped out into the 5 am darkness of San Francisco. As I watched my breath come out in cold, billowy clouds, I reminded myself that the success rates were higher for people who worked out in the morning. Squeezing my fingers together for warmth, I thought about how I was moving my health to the top of my priority list—and I set out walking.

It was October 1996 and my first attempt at exercising outside after a month of spending two days a week on the treadmill. I was about to be taught the difference between working out inside versus outside. Inside, the belt on the treadmill helps you regulate your pace, but on the pavement, you propel yourself. On this particular morning, I only lasted 15 minutes. I laugh when I look back on it now, but on that day, I was so discouraged. Returning home, my heavy men's size XXL sweats dripped with sweat, my face was red from the cold, and I was huffing and puffing in a desperate attempt to get the air I needed. What happened to all the progress I had made on the treadmill? Great. I'm moving backwards, not forward!

The next day, I was so sore, much more so than on the treadmill and my shins *killed me!* I thought, that's it, I can't do this. It's too much. After all, I'm sore so I must be hurting myself.

All these emotions were real and meant something to me at the time. What I couldn't see until later was that actually moving outside to work out not only was a new commitment, but it was a step forward and it was *progress.*

mind　body　spirit

The next five or six times I went out, it was not as bad. I was able to regulate my breathing and taste a little success. I went online and talked to other Connectors who had been there. They said, Tawni, that pain in your shins is normal. Tawni, I felt like quitting after the first time, too, but I kept at it, and I'm so glad I did.

In life there is always a time where we have to start something new. Whether it is a new job, a new city, or a new fitness lifestyle, it's not easy. Our brains try to figure out a million reasons why we shouldn't have made the move, why the old job was better, or why it would just be easier to stay wrapped in the warm bed covers. Luckily, the great thing about exercise is you feel instant gratification. You feel better when you're done. For me, working out made me proud of myself for the first time in my life. Here was something I wasn't doing because someone else told me to or gave me a paycheck to do, but because I was doing it for *me*.

When I moved my workouts outside, I tasted success, but not consistency. People still ask me all the time, how do you do it every day? How do you *keep* doing it? The consistency is the hardest part next to starting.

When I started changing my lifestyle in September 1996, I was not a morning person, so I just walked on the treadmill when it was convenient to me. I was working out after work—see how work came first? If I was going to go out to dinner, I certainly couldn't eat healthy—see what an easy lie that is? I cemented the foundation of my beginning when I heard Bob Greene speak at a book signing in Menlo Park, CA.

Looking back, I went to that signing hoping for an "excuse note." Remember when your Mom would write you a note excusing you from class because you were sick or had to go on a trip or something like that? That's what I was searching for from Bob Greene, whose role as a fitness guru was planted firmly in my mind, not just by his credentials but by Oprah's faith in him as well. I thought that if he heard all the stuff I had to do, maybe he would tell me, "Tawni, you're too busy, you can't exercise. You have no time."

When the woman next to me at the signing stood up to ask him a question, she explained that she commuted one hour to work each way every day and that she had to take her kids to various lessons and activities, etc. And I stood there thinking, "Yeah, see? She's too busy, just like I am. What do you have to say about that, Bob?"

Very politely, but very firmly, Bob told her that exercise was clearly not a priority in her life right now. That was a light bulb moment for me! Here I had driven to this bookstore looking for another way out, hoping that I could somehow get this man to tell me that I was so special that I could cop out. What happened instead is that I had this great realization. When you really *are* ready, this lifestyle will become a priority and everything else will fall into place behind it. I asked myself, what if my health was the most important thing in my life? At that moment, my attitude evolved to the point I needed it to and I never looked back. For me, that was as good as the construction workers pouring the cement for the bottom of the house because I was ready to build!

The changes I made in my life were tangible. I set two alarm clocks. I forced myself to go to bed earlier. Before I would stay up until eleven at night having drinks with clients. Even though it was hard for me to appear in public because of my embarrassment at how I looked, I rationalized it by telling myself it was "for work." Now my priority was getting up early the next morning to work out. I had always attended a lot of networking meetings for my job. I stopped going to those. Did I get support from my co-workers? Think again. My boss labeled me as "difficult" when I told him I wasn't attending those meetings because of my early morning date with myself.

But you know something happens mentally when you start making good decisions for you. When I got to the point where I was walking five days a week consistently, the scale rewarded me, but more importantly, I felt better. I made better food choices. My life turned around, the skies were clear and the wind was at my back.

So how do you take that first step? I mean, literally, whether it's out your front door, on to the treadmill, or into the car on your way to a nearby track—how do you start moving? There are several things you can do before you get your body moving.

Your focus

Have clearly in your mind *why* you are doing this. You aren't being bullied into this; you aren't being forced by someone else's idea of what your life should be. *You* are making the best decision for yourself and that is the glowing neon sign that should come up in your head whenever there's any doubt. This is about making the decision to put yourself and your health first.

mind 🏃 body 🏃 spirit 🏃

A lot of Connectors tell me that they work out so that they can see their grandchildren grow up. Others say it is because they want to have more energy for their kids. I have heard all kinds of goals from fitting into a wardrobe of nothing but size 8 to running a marathon to even   ing a better sex life! Sometimes it's a combination of lots of small goals with a larger picture of the desire for good health. Whatever gets you out there and keeps you out there—do what works for you.

One of the best things I did to maintain my focus was to create something I called an "I-can." Cutting out zillions of pictures of eyes from magazines, I pasted them all over an old coffee can. Each time I worked out, I put money in the "I-can," rewarding myself later with what accumulated in there. I gave new meaning to *earning* that money.

Changing habits

Life is daily. Daily choices. Daily decisions. When you make a decision, you are deciding what your priorities are. And when you make better choices for yourself, you gain self-confidence and continue to make better decisions. When you make certain choices, you will see that you are actually changing your habits.

Habits are powerful—whether they are good or bad. I just kept forming better and better habits and I still work on the habits that aren't getting me to where I want to go. It's an ongoing thing. All part of the journey. During the last three plus years, I have changed many habits and I'm still making discoveries along the way because *there is no finish line.*

What are your habits? How are you changing them? If you want different results, you need to think differently and take different actions. Your different thoughts, different choices and persistence will get you to your big goal.

Support from friends & family

People are social creatures by nature, so the idea of working out with someone else, having a little company as you greet the new day, is a welcome one. I encourage it because I think there can definitely be strength in numbers. The only challenge to this is when your friend cancels and it becomes that much easier for you to shrug off your workout for the day. Naturally, you had these expectations that you would be walking with your friend, together in your fitness quest. Now her kid's sick and you're all alone. What to do?

Since my health and fitness are mine and no one else's, I work out alone. Yes, it's lonely and yes it's tough to be motivated sometimes, but I do it because that's who I am. On weekends, I love getting together to run with local Connectors. During the week, it's just me, baby, pounding the sidewalks and the only company I have is my thoughts. Which I enjoy, actually. That's my time to clear out the cobwebs. That's how I like to look at it. That way, it stays a "get to," not a "have to."

Expect weird looks and perhaps some grumbling as that front door swings wide at 5 am and you vanish through it. Don't forget those mental flowers. Mine for this is, "I respect my body enough to want to take care of it." And that's totally about *me*. I'm not looking for approval anymore, except from myself.

I came back from a visit at my sister's house where I spent the weekend hiking (a great workout for your butt and quad muscles) and running along a river and up into the hills. The trees smelled as inviting as the campfire breakfast. My sister was talking with a group of her friends and commented to them "how afraid Tawni used to be all the time to try anything new." She turned to me and asked, "Why do you think you're not afraid anymore?"

I thought for a minute and said, "I think it's because I'm fit now. I have confidence in my body and its abilities." And my sister smiled and said, "Well, it's about damn time!" Later she introduced me as her sister, Tawni, a marathon runner. Who would have thought three years ago I would be thought of as a runner, much less a *marathon* runner? More like, here's my fat sister who is afraid to do anything but sit on her butt and eat herself to death!

Support like this from your family and friends can be a terrific motivator. So can working out with a partner. So can the ongoing support from the Connectors. But the real motivation has to come from inside. It's your own commitment that will make this work. You can do it, and you have to *believe* that you can do it. You can derail that destructive lifestyle train you have been riding for so long. You can choose a new way of living.

Consult a physician

Most people say this, but here's why it is so significant. If you are severely overweight, you'll feel better if you consult a physician before starting

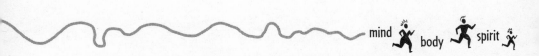

mind   body   spirit

any fitness program. I always think it is better to have more information about yourself than less. This will also help you to set some small goals.

If you aren't severely overweight, say you are 10 or 20 pounds overweight, it can still be a good starting point for you to chat with a physician, especially if you either haven't been physically active in years or have never been active.

I also like to funnel people who have a history of heart problems or other serious diseases to a physician before starting to work out because the information you can get from a physician can often dispel any preconceived fears you might be harboring. There is an activity level for everyone, but no two activity levels are the same.

As a general rule, if you're 35 or under and healthy, you probably don't need to consult a physician before you start to work out. But if you are older than 35 and have been pretty sedentary, I would recommend at least touching base with a physician.

Physicians don't know it all, but they can be a guide for your activity level when you are first beginning. Having the right information can help you avoid frustrating injuries and physical setbacks along your path to fitness.

Taking the leap

If you're just trying to get off the couch, plan your workout for any time that you can. If you're not a morning person, morning workouts may have to be something you work your way into. Incorporate your workout into your daily schedule. That is the key to making it part of your life forever. It can be as simple as walking on the treadmill while watching television. I would often come home from work and get on the treadmill.

And if you hear yourself say, "I don't feel like it," join the club. How often do we have to do things in life that we don't feel like doing? Every day! Do we really feel like going to the grocery store, paying bills, standing in line at the post office, or waking up at 2 am to feed the baby? So, do we feel like it? Irrelevant. Do we know we'll feel better after we do it? Definitely.

Of course, leave yourself open to use any trick you need to stay focused on your goal, no matter how small it may be. No one feels like working out, so lose this as an excuse (it's the best and most used one out there). I tell myself that I feel better when I walk 15 minutes a day. Or I feel better and have more energy for the whole day when I get out and knock down those first few miles.

One trick that works really well is to say to yourself, "It's only ten minutes. Just walk slowly. No pressure." Then once you are out there, you feel your mind dragging your body further than they both thought you would go.

I used to think, "I'll just walk to the bagel shop and back." That way, I was mentally thinking that I was just getting breakfast and not really working out. It lightened the mental load of "having" to work out. After three or four weeks, you'll find yourself having to use fewer and fewer tricks because it will become an ingrained habit for you.

Scheduling challenges

This is one of the strongest arguments for the morning workout and the one that kills the old "I'll do it later" theory. If you roll out of bed and get out the door, it's over with for the whole day. Do it before the kids get up, before your husband goes to work, and before you allow anything else to get in the way. A little tip: going to bed at a decent time makes it that much easier to get up the next morning.

I have known Connectors who are so busy that when they first started, all they could do was park the car as far away at possible at the mall or wherever they were running their errands. At least that forced them to move!

Carve out 15 or 20 minutes of your day—*somewhere*. Begin slowly and give yourself lots of encouragement. Each time you get out there and make the time for your fitness, pat yourself on the back and know that you're doing the best you can for you.

Exercise equipment such as treadmills, stationary cycles, stair steppers, etc. can work very effectively for people with harried schedules and for those of you who live in lousy weather. (I'll talk more about the pros and cons of various types of exercise equipment in the next chapter.)

Work

We all have horror stories and tales to tell about how work interferes with our lives, and not just our workouts. When I worked in the corporate world, I certainly had my share of success and won awards and stuff like that. And it was great. But none of that, none of the bonus checks or awards I received, can remotely compare to the feeling I get when I cross the finish line of a marathon or run the final steps of a long training run. Nobody could have told me that three years ago. I would have laughed in someone's face if they had told me I would be running 26.2 miles!

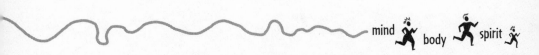

mind 🏃 body 🏃 spirit 🏃

Now I would be lying if I said I didn't miss the money. I do. But I recognize that the long hours and constant strain to make the money is a sacrifice. I had to meet with people and be available at all hours in order to accommodate customers and expand my clientele. But I have learned that some things are priceless (like my health, my peace of mind, and my personal time) and setting a big goal like fitness and health and working hard every day to achieve it has no price tag.

I saw the article in RW and at the time I had been in a running slump for a couple of years, running on and off, but with no consistency. The reason was I couldn't figure out how was I going to do my AM outside runs that I did four times a week for what seemed forever, because my husband left when my daughter was 2 1/2 (she just turned 6).

Of course, I couldn't leave my daughter for my morning runs. I decided to purchase a treadmill and at first was very enthusiastic about that, but that faded away as well. Then I got this issue of RW that hit me like a ton of bricks. It had to do with this girl with such contagious energy named Tawni, Connectors from all walks of life and "no more excuses." I was hooked.

The next day I signed on, told a handful of friends about the site, I put a change of running clothes in my car and every time I was visiting family or friends, I asked them for half an hour or so to run while they watched my daughter. I started doing whatever it took to "get out there." I also joined a gym at lunchtime and now the stressful days are less stressful and I have a schedule. I always took the freedom to run outside for granted.

What I realized through this experience is that if you want something bad enough you can get it, and the struggle makes the rewards sweeter. DONNA, CONNECTING IN NJ

We have all heard some famous, well-to-do person, suffering from some disease or affliction, say "I would give anything to have my health back." But, you see, even all their money could not help them in the end.

When I was working, work consumed me. Work was my priority above all else because of the money. But I lost vital parts of myself. I lost my health, I was very unfit, and quite frankly, I was not happy. But don't misunderstand, I am aware of people who have been able to structure their lives in a way that enables them to work, make plenty of money, and attend to themselves. They work out regularly, they are careful about what they eat, and they have managed to balance their lives. But they have figured out

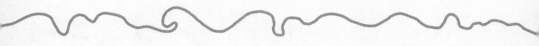

how to make this happen for themselves. For many of us, this may not be entirely possible. Something must give.

First, I made a list of all my excuses for not exercising. Then, for each excuse, I list-ed physical activities and places I could do those activities whenever I came up with that particular excuse. Some of my excuses were: it's too cold, it's too dark, it's too late, it's raining, I'm too tired, I don't have time to shower afterwards, I exercised extra yesterday, I don't want to go out again after work, I have class, the gym parking lot is too crowded, the treadmills are always taken, the gym isn't open on Saturday, I don't feel like getting up early on weekends, etc.

When it was cold, dark, or rainy I could walk on the treadmill or at the mall. When I went to the mall to buy something or to see a movie, I told myself I had to walk 3 laps around the inside of the mall (2 miles) before I could go in the store. When it was late or I was tired, I could walk up and down the stairs outside my apartment or inside the school building. When I didn't have time to shower after exercising, I could walk at a lower exertion level. When I had class after work, I could go to the gym before work or after class.

When I exercised extra the day before, I reminded myself that extra did not take the place of today and not exercising today made it easier not to exercise tomorrow. I routinely took my exercise clothes and shoes with me so I did not have to come home before going to exercise. When the gym parking lot was crowded I could walk to the gym; it was only about 3 blocks from my apartment. FLORENCE, CONNECTING IN CA

For me, for my own personal circumstances, I needed to cut out a certain amount of time from my work to make money to work on myself, my health, and my personal needs. You will have to evaluate your own situation to make a balance. Obviously, most of us can't just quit working. I'm not saying you should. What I *am* saying is try not to allow work to be an excuse for not working on yourself. Try not to allow work to prevent you from exercising and eating properly and maintaining the right attitude to live a healthy, happy life.

Understanding the basics

The decision to make regular exercise a part of your life is the crucial first step. Once you're there, though, you need to understand some basics about *how* to exercise so you derive the most benefit from your effort and keep yourself as injury-free as possible.

Stretching

Many people who enthusiastically dive into a new exercise program make the same mistake—they don't bother to stretch before and after their workouts. Why do you need to stretch? Well, stretching before your workout primes your muscles for activity, while stretching after your workout improves your flexibility and gives your muscles a way to cool down. When you work out, your muscles tend to tighten or constrict. If you don't warm up and then stretch, you are opening yourself up to a greater possibility for injury. In addition, you limit your muscles' range of motion over time. Overall, I recommend warming up and cooling down with anywhere from 5 to 15 minutes of stretching.

I do a little very light stretching right before my walk or run and then more extensive stretching immediately after. If I wake up at 5 am and I'm getting ready for a run, I naturally stretch my arms over my head before I even get out of my warm bed. That's a good place to start.

Before I stretch, I like to walk around for about five minutes so my body becomes a little more limber. After that, I stop and stretch. This acts the same way that preheating an oven does; it helps shake off that early morning stiffness and makes you less prone to injury when you stretch.

Just before you step out the door or begin your workout, you can start with some very simple stretches for legs and arms. I can get side aches really easily when I run, so I start by raising my arms straight over my head, standing tall, and breathing deeply. That gets more air into my diaphragm. I also stretch to the left and right sides, bending slightly at the waist and breathing deeply. I'm basically waking my body up to the idea that I'm about to work out.

When you do your leg stretches, you want to be sure not to *bounce* on your legs. A more static type of stretching is safer and not likely to injure or strain you. Here are the leg stretches I use; they work all the major muscles.

Quadriceps: Stand with your back straight and one arm on a wall or other solid object to brace yourself. Lift your left leg (you can cheat by using your hand to pull your foot up) and tuck your foot behind your thigh. Do this gently. Your knee should be pointing straight down at the ground and you should feel a slight tug in the front of your thigh. Hold for five seconds and repeat on the other leg.

Hamstring: Lie on the floor with your knees bent. Grab one leg with your hands just below your knee and let the opposite leg just remain in a relaxed bent position. Gently pull the leg you are holding in toward your chest and hold it that way for up to ten seconds. You should feel a tension in the back of the bent leg. Repeat this for the other leg.

Groin/Inner thighs: Sit on the floor and place the soles of your feet together. You can start with your feet extended slightly in front of you. Slowly allow your knees to drop toward the ground and at the same time scoot your feet toward you. You will feel tension in your groin and inside thigh area. When you first begin doing this stretch, you may keep your back straight; later as you increase your flexibility, you can lean forward for added stretching.

Achilles: You can stretch your Achilles tendon (located in the lower part of the back of your leg) with any curb or stair. Balance yourself against the wall if you have to. Stand on the front part (the balls) of your feet and keeping your legs and back straight, drop your heels down slowly and hold that for up to ten seconds. Be careful not to bounce!

Calf: Stand with your feet about shoulder width apart (comfortably) and parallel to each other. Bend your knees and lower your body, keeping your back straight, until you feel a stretching sensation in your calves. Hold this for at least five seconds.

Ankle: I find that by rotating my feet in clockwise and counter-clockwise circles, it helps avoid some of the stiffness you can get in your ankles from repetitive use. You can do this sitting down, too. Just extend your leg out so your foot is off the ground and rotate your foot only. Repeat for both feet.

Foot: Because of the motion you use in walking and running, I like to stretch my feet in this simple way. While standing with both feet approximately shoulder width apart, extend one leg behind you and lift your foot so only the toes are touching the ground. Repeat for the other foot. This has helped me a lot with foot cramps!

Breathing

You probably don't think about it much right now, but proper breathing will become very important to you as your activity level increases. If you have never run before, you may not know that runners tend to breathe

mind body spirit

predominantly through their mouths. Why? Arguably, this is the best way to get the most air into your lungs. And you need to know about breathing because as you start to work out more and more, breathing is crucial.

Running makes you short of breath. So what can you do? Pay attention to your breathing. Even when you are walking this is important. Listen to yourself breathe in and out as you walk or run. Adjust your breathing to match your speed.

Deeper, longer breaths not only relax your body, which makes side aches less likely, but also give your body the oxygen it needs.

Water

When you exercise aerobically (and I'll get to the importance of aerobic exercise next), your body gets hotter and hotter. That's why you start to sweat—your body is trying its best to cool you down. However, you need to replace the fluids you sweat off or you'll see a definite decrease in your performance. In the early days when I didn't have enough water in my system, I really suffered from side aches and general fatigue. Fortunately that's not a problem for me anymore (just call me the water girl), but I had to learn it the hard way.

But don't just drink water when you exercise. Ideally, you should drink about 64 ounces (2 quarts) of water a day (preferably bottled or filtered).

You may not need water when you are only walking for 15 minutes or less, but it's not a bad habit to get into the habit of carrying water with you. There are all kinds of reasons, but the most important one is that as you condition your body, you will lower your "sweat threshold—the point at which you begin to sweat. In other words, the better shape you're in, the faster you will start to sweat because your body has become more efficient. Therefore, your body will demand water and/or a replacement of the fluids it loses during your workout. Water helps the overall performance of your muscles and the delivery of oxygen throughout your body. It can help you avoid that feeling of muscle fatigue that can really slow your workout down.

When you build up your endurance so that you're walking more briskly for longer distances or even running, you especially need water. No matter what the weather is, exercise can quickly deplete your fluid levels. For long runs or walks, carry a pack or water bottle and sip it slowly about every 15 minutes.

Keep in mind that if you are a soft drink freak, like I was before I weaned myself off of it, even though you may be drinking a lot of water, it gets literally "leached" out of your body by the caffeine. All the water you are pouring in can only stay there if your body becomes accustomed to having that much fluid. You'll be able to visually monitor how hydrated you are by the color of your urine. Sounds crazy, but it's true! When you are getting enough liquids, your urine will be clear or pale yellow. When you first start drinking water consistently, you may find yourself running to the bathroom just about every five minutes! Don't worry; it will pass as your body "learns" to absorb what it needs and gets rid of the rest.

Benefits of Water

· Can suppress appetite

· Helps your body metabolize stored fat by flushing out your liver and kidneys

· Relieves fluid retention problems (that bloated feeling)

· Flushes out unwanted salt from your system

· Helps maintain muscle tone

Aerobic exercise

You hear people talk about exercising aerobically but what does it mean? The word aerobic means "with oxygen." Why is that important? An aerobic exercise is a workout in which your volume of breathing (the amount of air you take in to your body) is increased and your heart is forced to beat faster than usual for a prolonged period of time. The result is an increased amount of oxygen-rich blood to the muscles you are using. Aerobic exercises such as running, walking, water fitness, cycling, jumping rope, aerobics classes, cross-country skiing and dancing can strengthen your heart and lungs. How? By distributing more oxygen throughout your whole body and by enabling the most important muscle you have in your body—your heart—to work more efficiently. Aerobic exercise makes you stronger and, in a sense, you become more durable.

Aerobic exercise is also the most *efficient* way to burn fat. "Stop and start" activities like baseball, golf, bowling, etc. are wonderful, but they are not considered aerobic because you are not constantly maintaining an accelerated heart rate for an extended time period.

Experts recommend that you engage in at least three aerobic sessions per week of 20 minutes each. Set that as a big goal for those of you just starting out. Eventually, you will want to increase the amount of time you work out although not necessarily the intensity of your workout.

mind body spirit

Measuring your aerobic level

Probably the most accurate way to measure your aerobic level is your heart rate. I have included a chart here to help you figure out where your heart rate should be during your workout. To get the most health benefits from aerobic activity, you should exercise at a level strenuous enough to raise your heart rate to your target. Your target heart rate is 50 to 75 percent of your maximum heart rate (maximum means the fastest your heart can beat). Your target is the category closest to your age. For example, a 35-year-old's target heart rate is 93-138 beats per minute.

If your heart is beating faster than your target heart rate, you are working too hard—slow down. If your heart is beating slower than your target heart rate, challenge yourself to work a little harder. When you first begin exercising, aim for the lower part of your target (50 percent). As you reach more and more of your baby goals and get into better shape, you can gradually reach the higher part of your target (75 percent). Above all, exercise at a pace that is comfortable for you. As you become more conditioned, you will feel more comfortable exercising and can slowly increase your intensity level.

Age	Target Heart Rate Zone 50-75%	Average Maximum Heart Rate 100%
20-30 years	98-146 beats per min.	195
31-40 years	93-138 beats per min.	185
41-50 years	88-131 beats per min.	175
51-60 years	83-123 beats per min.	165
61+ years	78-116 beats per min	155

NIH PUBLICATION NO. 96-4031, APRIL 1996

Another good indicator of your aerobic level is the speaking test. The speaking test is something you do as you are working out. Let's say that it takes about 10 minutes to get warmed up while you are engaged in some aerobic activity. You should be able to carry on brief conversation without gasping to know that you are at the right intensity level.

Metabolism

I find that this is a mystery word for many people I talk to. Metabolism is basically the amount of energy (read: calories) your body burns to stay in operation. It's always running, kind of like your refrigerator, just humming away. The change in how fast or slow your metabolism hums is related to your body composition; in other words, how much muscle you have as opposed to how much fat.

While aerobic exercise burns fat and calories, the best way to rev your metabolism is strength training (more about my own strength training routine in the next chapter). The reason is that the more toned muscle you have, the more your body draws on fat stores. This is another reason that dieting doesn't work because when you diet you lose not just fat but muscle as well, meaning you're actually slowing your metabolism. Depriving your body of food by eating low-calorie "diets" instead of making balanced food choices sends the message to your body that you're starving—your metabolism reacts by slowing down its rate of burning calories, conserving them in a survival mode.

Obviously building muscle through strength training is only one aspect in changing your weight and metabolism; you need to combine it with a change in your food choices and aerobic exercise in order to see a difference in your body.

PULSE

Take your pulse as you are still exercising for most accurate results. Place your fingers on your wrist just below the palm of your hand (or right below your jaw); you'll feel your pulse there. While looking at a watch, count the number of pulse beats over six seconds. Multiply that by ten and you'll know your heart rate per minute.

Getting the right gear

While you need the basics—shoes and clothes appropriate for the weather—to begin, you don't have to go out and buy a whole wardrobe of clothes, shoes, heart monitors, watches, and hats before you start working out. For a lot of people, gearing up happens gradually. They start with the basics and bit by bit, as they get into fitness more and more, they *want* all the "foo-foo" that goes with it. The accessories are more important to some people than others, but what will most likely happen is that you too will start with shoes and a few workout clothes and eventually add accessories and equipment.

Shoes

When you start working out, you will realize that your feet are the center of the universe. They need the support and cushioning that a sturdy, properly fitting pair of shoes bring.

Whether you're walking or running, go to a specialty running store where they know about shoes and will look at each individual's foot needs separately. I won't name names, but we've all been inside those bewildering, huge warehouse-type stores that carry every piece of sporting equipment

mind body spirit

known to man. And guess what? The people that work there aren't specialists. And you *need* a specialist because *you* are special.

When I was looking for the right shoes for me, I went to a specialty running store that I got out of the back of *Runner's World*. I must have tried on a dozen pairs of running shoes that day. I walked in them, ran in them, put my bare, wet foot down on a piece of paper to see my foot type—let's put it this way: I was there for a while. They say there are two things you don't want hurting in life: your teeth and your feet. And that is definitely true!

· Nine out of ten women are wearing shoes that are too small for their feet
· Eight out of ten women say their shoes are painful
· Women are nine times more likely to develop a foot problem because of improper fitting shoes than a man

AMERICAN ACADEMY OF ORTHOPAEDIC SURGEONS, NATIONAL SHOE RETAILERS ASSOCIATION

Bring a pair of socks the weight that you would walk or run in; this affects the fit of the shoes. Take your time and make sure you are absolutely comfortable in the pair of shoes you select. You don't have to spend a lot of money to get a decent pair of shoes; I would stay in the $75 to $100 range to start. Pay attention to how the shoe feels, not what it looks like, whose name is on it, whether there is leather or nylon on the top, or what kind of footprint it leaves. Believe me, you don't even think about that type of stuff when you are working out.

When you get to the store, have them measure your feet and don't be shocked when they bring out a pair of shoes that is a half or a whole size larger than your dress shoes. When you run, your feet swell and you really don't want your toes jammed up against the front of the shoes.

Know that sometimes the pair that feels okay in the store doesn't always work the same way when you run in them. But that's life; there are no guarantees. The nice thing is that once you find a pair you like, you can order it from a catalog like Roadrunner Sports (www.roadrunnersports.com) and they guarantee the shoes and other items that they sell. If your feet (or other body parts) change within two months of buying the shoes, you can send them back.

Don't be tempted to dry your shoes on the air vent after you come back from a walk or run in the rain; it cracks the rubber and shortens the life of the shoes. Plan to replace your workout shoes every three to five months, depending on the amount you exercise each week. If you're running or walking, 300 to 500 miles is a good gauge (that's why it's great to have a log to keep track of such big numbers!).

Clothes

I was living in Burlingame, CA and I wanted to get new exercise clothes. When I first began working out (mostly walking and running), I didn't know that there were plus sizes available for women so I was walking and running in 100 percent cotton men's sweats and cotton doesn't breathe, let me tell you! I had heard of this new fabric called Coolmax that wicks sweat away from your body. I thought, "With the way you sweat, honey, you should buy stock in this company!"

I knew there was a runner's store near where I kept a post office box, but when I asked the postal employee where it was and she told me, I couldn't believe it. I had driven by there a million times, but I hadn't seen it. Guess that shows you only see what you want to see, because when I went looking for it, it was obvious.

The first time I went in there were too many people in the store. I was embarrassed and I left. The second time, the owner of the store helped me. Shawn looks like a typical runner: tall, thin, muscular. She was extremely supportive and encouraging, and best of all, I got the fabric I wanted.

Now I know that there is a catalog called Junonia (www.junonia.com) that specializes in workout clothing for large women. I also have bought things from Champion and from Moving Comfort. In fact, Moving Comfort has a large-size product line that is in development.

You also need a good bra. Let's dispel a myth. Your breasts don't sag because you aren't wearing a bra; they sag because of the amount of fatty tissue inside of them. And most women I know don't like wearing bras because they're uncomfortable. But let me tell you, you need a bra when you're working out. Not just for the simple fact that you want those things secure and not knocking you out, but it just feels better! If you are well endowed in the chest region, try the Frogbra from Title 9 Sports, a mail order catalog by and for women.

Now that I have found Coolmax, I don't like to work out in anything that doesn't have it and that includes exercise bras. Buy a bra that is comfortable and holds you securely, but doesn't make you gasp for air. When you go to try one on, start with a size slightly larger than you would normally wear in an underwire or other type of bra. Remember, fitness is about movement and if you can't breathe when you move or if the bra chafes you too badly, it can be not only painful but discouraging.

mind body spirit

Above all, the clothes you wear to work out in should be loose and comfortable. While your shoes are the most important, having a nice, cute outfit can be an incentive to work out. Buying new workout clothes can also be a reward for goals achieved.

I hate shorts riding up my butt, so I have traditionally always worn long running tights, you know, the spandex-y, Coolmax material that stretches all the way to your ankle. I have found that bike shorts can really help with chafing and rubbing between your thighs because they tend to keep your legs farther apart.

Dressing for the weather

When you walk or run in the winter, your most challenging months for exercise as far as I'm concerned because no one likes to be freezing cold, make sure you go out prepared. Although you can expect to be slightly cold when you start out, the walking or running will warm you up.

I wear running tights, a long sleeve Coolmax shirt, and if it's really crazy or raining out, a jacket like Clima-Fit or Storm-Fit by Nike. These are waterproof and wind resistant, but light enough to work out in. Nike is not the only brand out there that makes this type of jacket; check the Roadrunner Sports catalog for more options on jackets. I also wear a fleece cap with earflaps to protect my ears from the wind, as well as gloves so my fingers won't snap off from the cold.

When it's cold out, one of the first places you lose heat is through your head. That's where that wonderful fleece cap comes in. However, if you start to feel like you're boiling water under there, your cap is the first thing to remove to let a little heat escape.

Generally, I find that if I'm not cold for the first 10 minutes of my run, I am dressed too warmly and will probably be too hot later in the run. And not only that, I will feel more dehydrated, too. So try dressing for sweating. In other words, it's normal to feel a little chilly when you start out, but your body will warm you up as you exercise aerobically. You may find that you start out with a few layers and that your top layer is one that you can unzip and let off some of the heat that you generate.

Fitness accessories

As I think back over my experience with walking and then running, there are some things that I wish I had known when I started out. One of them is how to avoid blisters and chafing on all parts of my body. I tried taping my toes and I also tried Vaseline (I *hated* getting this on my fingers), but now the way I deal with any kind of irritation that comes from working out is Body Glide (www.sternoff.com).

Body Glide is a product that is non-greasy and glides on like you put on your deodorant. For me it's been a godsend! I put it on my feet, under my bra, between my thighs—I'm telling you, there's no place it can't help! Since I have been putting it on my feet, I haven't had blisters.

The other half of the non-blistering feet connection is Thor-Lo socks. These are socks that have—you guessed it—Coolmax in them. You can get running or walking socks in many different lengths, materials, and thickness, but for me, thin works best. You'll find Thor-Lo socks and other Coolmax brands at your local specialty running store or online at Roadrunner Sports.

For runs over six miles, I use a water carrier called the Ultimate Pack. It doesn't flop around like those other annoying carriers because you can really cinch it tightly, either in front or in back. It's also curved so it fits you more naturally. The side pouches are also great for carrying granola bars, power gels, keys, and cell phones.

What about heart monitors? Some people say you should have a heart monitor to measure your intensity level. A heart monitor is an electronic device that you either strap to your arm or across your chest to keep track of your heart rate. You program the monitor to alert you with a beep to let you know when you are working out too slowly or too hard. I do use a heart rate monitor made by Polar, although I don't use it all the time. Unless your doctor tells you that you need to monitor your heart rate carefully, I personally don't think that you need one. A good monitor could easily cost $100, but the sweat and speaking test can help you achieve the same end.

Fitness kick-start tips

In the next chapter, I give you specific recommendations for starting and developing a fitness program, including several activities you can try when you're a beginner and more advanced workouts you can try once your endurance and conditioning levels increase. For now, here are my 10 fitness kick-start tips to help get you on the road to fitness, health, and happiness.

mind body spirit

1 **Make a decision for life.** Remember: you get started only when you have decided to make fitness a regular part of our life. Consistency is critical for success.

2 **Maintain focus.** Do this by making a daily recommitment to yourself (no one else), and adopt my "I-can" attitude.

3 **Get support.** Try to find someone to either work out with you or to become your fan for ongoing support. For some of us, becoming a Connector is our only real source of support. Join us now at the www.connectingconnectors.com web site.

4 **Reschedule your life.** Work around your fitness routine. Find reasons to *make* this happen, not excuses not to.

5 **Get the proper tools.** You have heard it said that you need the right tools to get the job done. Well, in this case, the right tools means the right shoes, clothes, equipment, whatever, to make fitness part of your life.

6 **Get aerobic.** Learn what it means to be aerobic, choose aerobic activities, and pay attention to your breathing.

7 **Avoid injuries.** Learn about stretching and other basic injury-avoidance techniques.

8 **Drink water.** Learn about the benefits of water.

9 **Develop an overall interest in fitness.** Try to be open to new experiences, such as different forms of aerobic activity, even if you are not ready to engage in the activity right away. Read up on products and techniques, and check out new web sites.

10 **Start now!** Do something now, today, to get you going. The sooner your start, the sooner you will experience results, the sooner your life will change. I promise. NO MORE EXCUSES!

I hear lots of people tell me that the hardest thing for them is to start. I hope that the tips and tools I have shared with you in this chapter can help you on your own path to fitness. We have all been there. I like to challenge people in their thinking. Let me challenge you at this moment. What makes you think you *can't* begin a fitness program? Think about that as you plan your fitness routine in the next chapter.

Your own fitness routine

Overslept again this morning. Meant to go exercise but can't seem to get up in the morning, so I'll try and walk on the treadmill after I get done with all my sales calls. Of course who am I kidding? Half the time I never do it after work either. There's got to be an easier way. But I know deep down inside there isn't. If I want to be healthy and get below 200 pounds it's going to take work. I've really developed some bad habits with these crazy work hours and all the traveling back and forth.

Okay, tomorrow I'll commit to drinking a glass of water and walk 1 mile on the treadmill. My calves hurt every time I go all the way up to a mile. But I'm sure the more I do it the easier it will get. I wonder if I'll ever like exercising. Doubt it. I'd rather sleep in. But I suppose sleeping in isn't going to stop me from ripping out the seams in my skirts and staying below the 200-pound mark. I'll try to get up early tomorrow.

JOURNAL ENTRY, APRIL 18, 1996

Walking down the block and back a few times is fine at first, but now you want to establish a routine, to put some sort of structure into your workout plan. How often, how long, and how vigorously you exercise is something that only you can determine.

The right activity for you

When you start to craft your fitness routine, you'll want to blend several elements into your workouts. You will want an activity you enjoy. You'll also need to be aerobic, so that knocks out a few activities right away. Overall, you will want to take into consideration your background, age, goals, etc. Ask yourself these questions:

How physically fit are you? What do you hope to achieve by exercising? Do you see exercise as a social activity or something you do alone? Would you rather do the majority of your workouts in your house or outside? What activity will fit into your schedule the most easily?

Your personal workout routine

Your answers to those questions will help you develop your workout routine. Keep in mind what you want to accomplish and understand that

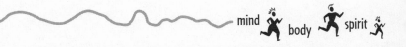

mind   body   spirit

everyone starts in a different place with a personal fitness plan. If you have been running for years, you are not going to be in the same shape as someone who has just started briskly walking three times a week.

Ideally, your fitness plan should include cardiovascular and muscular endurance activities, as well as muscular strength and flexibility exercises. What does all this mean?

I've been running every morning at 5am for about 13 years now—and never ONCE has it been easy to get up and do it. Thirteen years and never once! And I am definitely not someone who leaps out of bed every morning excited to get moving. Why do I keep doing it? It is the fastest, most efficient and effective way for me to keep my weight down—and I know that if I don't do it very first thing... it absolutely does not happen. I've tried telling myself, "Oh I'll feel better if I sleep in now, then run after work," but the plain fact is that by the time I get home from work the LAST thing I feel like doing is getting my running clothes on and hitting the streets.   INGRID, CONNECTING IN OR

Cardiovascular

"Cardio," as it is sometimes called, is how efficiently your body delivers oxygen and nutrients to tissues and removes waste. When I go out for a long run, my cardiovascular endurance is being tested because I am pushing my body for a length of time. You may find that, depending on your level of fitness, your heart beats quite rapidly when you work out. People who are in excellent physical shape have very slow heart rates. Why? Because their hearts don't have to work as hard to deliver the blood to various areas of the body; they have, in essence, conditioned their heart (which is a muscle after all) and made it strong. Aerobic exercise provides this cardiovascular workout.

Muscular endurance

This is the ability your muscles have to respond to long-term use, as in running. You can also test your muscular endurance by doing push-ups, which would be testing your arm and shoulder muscles. You are basically asking your muscles to repeat the same or similar movements over an extended period of time. This determines how long you will be able to work out at any given time.

Of course, muscle fatigue will occur when you press yourself beyond your current level of conditioning. Muscle soreness, which you may feel a couple of days after a workout, is simply a result of forcing your muscles to work harder than usual. But this is a good soreness. Eventually, the more you exercise and the longer you exercise during a given workout, the soreness goes away, and the less fatigue you feel. Beware, however, that dehydration will induce fatigue no matter how well conditioned you may be. This is why water is so important.

Flexibility

As I mentioned in the last chapter, stretching is essential for good muscle flexibility. Your level of flexibility means the amount that you are able to move joints and muscles through their full range of motion. I think of the old "can you touch your toes" test that kids like to do; that is a good measure of how flexible your back leg muscles are.

I like to do the flexibility part before and after my running or whatever workout I am doing that day. Up to 15 minutes of stretching, especially after your workout, is very beneficial for your muscles and can increase their ability to do what you want them to do!

Muscular strength

Measure this by the number of weight repetitions you can do comfortably. In this case you are using your muscles for a short amount of time. This would not only be the number of repetitions you can do, but, for example, also the amount of weight you can lift.

For example, walking, running, and cycling strengthen the muscles in your legs. You know you are getting stronger when doing hill work (going uphill and downhill) does not result in fatigue or soreness. Another sign of strength is the muscular definition you can actually see in your legs, particularly your quadriceps and calf muscles.

What do I start with?

I advocate walking for anyone who is just getting into fitness. It's easy to start, costs virtually nothing, and you can be anywhere to do it. After several weeks (or possibly months) of consistent walking, and particularly after you know you are able to increase your distance and speed comfortably, you may be ready to try an additional form of aerobic activity, such as jogging/running, cycling, skating, or water fitness.

mind body spirit

Now that I'm in shape, I run every other day at least 3 to 5 miles, usually longer on the weekends. I use the recumbent bike or the step equipment at the gym on the days that I don't run, and I lift weights 2 to 3 times a week. I also do a water workout, especially during injury times, and I cycle every couple of weeks. You can build up to this level too. But you have to start with baby steps.

Of course, there are other aerobic activities you can do, but I wanted to mention only those activities I personally enjoy doing regularly as part of my workout routine, and that I feel are the best. I suggest you try as many as you can, and from that you will determine what is best suited to your needs and requirements. Running will always be my first pick, but all these other activities are great, too.

Fewer than 10% of adults exercise at least four times a week and more than half quit within six months of starting an exercise program. The same problems hold true for children; only 32% of American children can pass a simple test of muscular strength, flexibility, and cardiovascular endurance.

WEBMD.COM (3/99)

Walking

A recent study of nearly 73,000 women done by the National Heart, Blood and Lung Institute confirms that just three hours of brisk walking a week can reduce the risk of heart disease 35 to 40 percent. And it's never too late to start. Women who were basically couch potatoes when the eight-year study began had the same reduction in risk of heart disease.

According to the National Sporting Goods Association, exercise walking grew 4.3 percent in 1996 to 73.3 million Americans. Walking is one of the most effective exercises for weight loss and overall health because you can walk regularly for long periods of time and not face the daunting injuries possible in running. Walking is a low-impact activity that you can do anytime, anyplace, and in any weather.

Walking is a great way to build endurance, especially if you are just starting out. I walked an entire year before ever running. Brisk walking is the key. This is subjective, but one example is if you're on a treadmill to shoot for 3 mph or more, or less than 20 minutes per mile. Unless you are coming from an active background, this is going to be challenging enough for you to begin with. Remember: what's important is that you are moving.

Now that you know how great a workout walking can be, where should you walk? I see a lot of people walking on the local high school or college track and I think in terms of safety, that is a great idea. The track surface is easy on your joints and you can measure your distance more easily than walking on the street. Of course, I also think you need to mix up track walking with some street walking or you'll go out of your mind with boredom!

A lot of parks have trails you can use and that can be a real treat for your mind and your eyes. Moving through trees is also cooler, and we all know that helps when you're getting aerobic!

The best exercises are not only aerobic, but also condition your heart and lungs. Walking can certainly meet these criteria, but don't fool yourself into thinking you're working out when you aren't.

For example, most people walking through a mall are not doing aerobic exercise. Wandering from store to store is not aerobic and does little or nothing for your heart and lungs. You stroll along, chat, look in windows, and stop off at different stores. But if you walk *briskly* through a mall for at least 15 minutes (preferably for 20 to 30 minutes) without stopping at any enticing shops, you can turn a mall trip into an aerobic activity. Mall walking is also a great "plan B" for cold, rainy or windy weather.

Once a week won't do it. However, if you walk briskly through the mall— heart rate elevated, breathing forcefully, and sweating—at least three times a week for up to 30 minutes, you're making good fitness strides.

I exercise at night because I NEED to get out of the house after being home with the tots all day! Needless to say, I don't need to talk myself into having some time for ME. I find running to be the best stress reliever! When I come home and shower after running I feel like I can do the whole day all over again, which is good because I have to the next day!   DEB, CONNECTING IN FL

Once you achieve a solid level of fitness with walking and are walking an hour or more two to three times a week, then you can focus on increasing the difficulty of your walks. Vary your walking workouts: walk faster, go further, or include hill workouts. Continue to vary the length of time and terrain of your walks to keep your workouts interesting and fresh. Measure several courses using your car odometer or the rule of 10 city blocks to a mile to measure different routes.

When I looked into walking, I discovered that walking has its own culture. There are walking clubs, races, meditation groups, special events (I'm

mind body spirit

sure you have heard about the various fund raising walking events), and various other organizations oriented towards walking. To make things interesting, many people incorporate rigorous hiking treks, sometimes in exotic places, like the Royal Incan Road hike, which is a five-day trek in the Peruvian Andes. Many others are content hiking in their local mountains (if there are any). For competitive types, racewalking is another way to stay fit and keep things interesting. I personally have never understood how to racewalk, but the Racewalking Foundation in Pasadena, CA (818-577-2264) offers plenty of material on how, where, and when.

Carolyn Scott Kortge, author of *The Spirited Walker,* combines fitness walking and meditation to make walking a mind, body, and soul exercise. *Walking* magazine is a great source of information on walking, interesting places to walk, product reviews, special walking events, and reviews of walking books. You can also get great information on all aspects of walking at the About.com web site (http://walking.miningco.com/sports/walking).

Walking is an exercise that works great and is accessible to everyone. You can see results fairly quickly and make great "strides" toward a healthier you. Walking should be the first type of aerobic activity that you do as you begin your regular commitment to fitness.

Jogging/Running

Jogging is just running very slowly. You may even try breaking up your walks with short periods of walk/jogs for two or three minutes at a time, returning to walking at a brisk sweat-inducing pace. Give yourself at least eight to nine weeks of longer and longer walk/run sessions. Then you may begin actually running exclusively, if running is your goal.

If I am training for a long race or doing a long run, I run five minutes and walk one minute. Or I vary it. I run nine minutes and walk one minute—whatever I can handle.

In October of 1998 I weighed 240 pounds and was a size 24. Miserable and depressed I had to do something, and I had to do it now! I started running at 240 pounds. It was hard. I couldn't run 10 yards without the feeling that I was going to die, but I kept at it. I changed my eating habits to fuel my runs, and I started to see the difference. As of today (July 24, 1999), I am a size 12! I have cut my size in half!   LYNN, CONNECTING IN IN

RUNNER'S WORLD 10-WEEK TRAINING PLAN

(Created by Budd Coates, Health Promotions Manager at Rodale Press)
www.runnersworld.com

Before you start with this schedule, get your legs ready with eight days of walking; walk for 20 minutes a day for the first four days, then increase to 30 minutes a day for four more days. Now you're ready to begin with week I.

Each week of the program, do your run/walk workouts on Monday, Wednesday, Friday, and Saturday, and take Tuesday, Thursday, and Sunday off.

10-WEEK TRAINING PLAN

WEEK 1	Run 2 minutes,	walk 4 minutes.	Repeat five times.
WEEK 2	Run 3 minutes,	walk 3 minutes.	Repeat five times.
WEEK 3	Run 5 minutes,	walk 2.5 minutes.	Repeat four times.
WEEK 4	Run 7 minutes,	walk 3 minutes	Repeat three times.
WEEK 5	Run 8 minutes,	walk 2 minutes.	Repeat three times.
WEEK 6	Run 9 minutes,	walk 2 minutes.	Repeat twice & run 8 min.
WEEK 7	Run 9 minutes,	walk 1 minute.	Repeat three times.
WEEK 8	Run 13 minutes,	walk 2 minutes.	Repeat twice.
WEEK 9	Run 14 minutes	walk 1 minute.	Repeat twice.
WEEK 10	Run 30 minutes.		

Now, there is no question that running is not for everyone. Running does take its toll. I still struggle with aches and pains with my knees, hips, and sometimes my legs. But running is definitely the most efficient workout for me: It does not take as long to do my workout, and I know that I'm stronger, my heart is stronger, and my lungs are stronger. I also have much more confidence in myself than ever before. So for me, it's worth it and I love to run.

I am often asked why I chose running as my ultimate workout. One of the best things about running is its immediate effect on your cardiovascular fitness. Although running is certainly one of the more difficult things to do consistently, it is also one of the fastest ways to see results, both in terms of overall fitness and in calorie burning.

mind body spirit

I also feel like a true athlete when I run. It does so much for my self-confidence and my self-esteem. When I can reach those baby goals on my way to a big goal, it is so good for my head. For example, being able to complete a 10K (6.2 miles) in less than an hour was such a high for me. No matter what, no one can take that accomplishment away from you; it comes from your effort and no one else's.

Another thing is that running can take you to so many interesting places. Whenever I am in a new city, I love to check out the running trails or great places for runners like along rivers or lakes. I see parts of the city that I wouldn't otherwise get to see.

The transition from walking to running

I had been walking on my treadmill and I found that I could no longer walk fast enough to keep my heart rate up where I needed it. But I assumed that I was too fat to run. I also assumed that if you were going to be a runner, you had to go out and run five miles right away. Then I discovered the beginning runner's program on *Runner's World* web site. That really unlocked my thinking.

I walked for eight weeks with no weight loss. I knew that I was strengthening my lower body so that I would not be injured when I began jogging. In those eight weeks my eating routine became more committed and my attitude improved. In the ninth week I started jogging. First, one minute jog with 5 minute walks. Eventually, I worked up to one mile jog and one minute walk. In week ten I lost 7 pounds and since then I have lost one pound a week.

On August 1, 1999, it will have been 6 months since I connected. I have lost 20 pounds so far, my longest run has been 6 miles in one hour, seven minutes. Once a week, I run intervals with Tawni at the local high school track. I do resistance training with a personal trainer at a gym two times a week. I cycled 85 miles last week with my wife and I have dropped almost 4 inches from my waist size. I bought new pants last month and now they are loose again. ANTHONY, CONNECTING IN CA

Cycling

Getting on a bicycle, either a road bike or a mountain bike, is something I do now and then to keep my workout routine interesting. What is greatly satisfying is that I can now actually get on a bike. Obviously when you are well over 200 pounds like I was, getting on a bike of any kind is not exactly an option. You know you are making progress if you can get on a bike and ride a few miles and feel great doing it.

Cycling can be one of those transition activities you do after you reach a certain level of conditioning. You give yourself that as a goal. It is well worth it. Once you begin riding, you may decide that it is an activity you want to include in your weekly routine. You will want to map out an area near where you live, taking into account the distance, terrain, convenience, safety, and other variables before venturing out.

I do outdoor cycling maybe every other week or so. I enjoy getting out and feeling the wind in my face. I also like the workout cycling gives me. When I first started out, I followed the fitness training recommendations made by a friend of mine, an experienced cyclist.

To start making cycling a part of your regular workout, first keep your rides to 20 to 30 minutes, three times per week and no more. You need to condition yourself. You can consider cycling to work, to the store, to the post office, wherever, to get out there and moving on your bike. Try to peddle briskly, but don't get out of breath. As you feel yourself getting stronger, try to cycle five days for 30 minutes each time out. But be careful not to increase the amount of time you ride by more than 10 percent per week. Condition yourself gradually.

Once you've built up your endurance, your weekly cycle workout can include one day per week of speed work, particularly if you are trying to firm your legs (muscle tone equals a more efficient metabolism which equals more efficient fat-burning). One day a week is enough since you are pushing yourself harder on that day than on your regular workout days. Remember riding too fast won't yield fat burning results, so peddle steadily and consistently without being out of breath. Also, on a speed day you don't have to ride far, just whatever distance you cover during a moderate 30 minute ride. You can build speed with short bursts of fast riding that last a couple of minutes followed by much slower recovery riding.

On the day after a speed work ride, you should take an easy day ride, the sort of ride you might take with family members or friends who aren't at the pace you are at during your regular workout. These easy days give your body a chance to refresh and actually strengthen itself for the more demanding days.

Also beware that it is easy to become dehydrated while cycling. As with running, make sure you have plenty of water or you will suffer from fatigue.

mind body spirit

What do you wear when you want to make outdoor cycling part of your regular workout? You'll soon discover that a cotton T-shirt and a pair of pants are too hot. And since bike seats are so often small and uncomfortable, I recommend bike shorts that are padded in the back to help cushion what we all refer to as your butt bone (coccyx in medical terms).

There are those people who argue that you get a better workout on a real bike versus a stationary bike. As far as I'm concerned, the stationary cycle is a tool of convenience. It can give you an aerobic workout, and even though stationary cycling is boring, you can at least read or watch TV. But when it's nice out, and you want to keep your workout routine interesting, I definitely encourage you to try outdoor biking. You could get yourself a road bike, like a 10 or 15 speed. But I think mountain biking is much more fun.

For those who are not familiar with mountain bikes, these are bikes with big tires and extra strong suspensions to withstand the pounding and riding on rough terrain. To get started you can get a beginner's bike for between $200 and $300, plus you will want to get a helmet for another $30 to $50.

Another benefit of outdoor cycling is that there is a whole culture around cycling, just as there is with walking and running. There are a whole slew of road/mountain bike clubs, races, tours, and various events to go to and share with other enthusiasts. It's lots of fun. You can go online and find an unbelievable number of web sites devoted to cycling. An especially good one for people just getting started is www.bikescape.com.

In early spring 1999 I went to help Bob Greene and Oprah kick off Bob's new book, *Keep the Connection,* by starting a nationwide bike trek. Oprah and I rode with Bob out of Long Beach, CA a few miles before he stopped to do a book signing at a bookstore in the area. It was a blast! Thousands of people showed up at the bike trek starting point.

Inline skating/Rollerblading

Skating can be a really fun aerobic activity, or terrifying, depending on your experience. Years ago, before the polyurethane single row of wheels attached to a shoe became known as the Rollerblade or inline skate, there were the steel, four-wheeled roller skates. Nearly everyone tried roller skates as a kid. But those days are long gone. The Rollerblade (which is the actual name of the product and the company that invented them) is what everyone is doing these days. And the fact is that in-line skating is considered to be nearly as aerobic as running. Apparently in-line skating gives your hips, thighs, and shins a greater workout than running or cycling. Also, because there is virtually no pounding while skating, in-line skating is considered a low-impact activity.

The trouble with in-line skating is that it takes some skill to learn to do it (you probably want to hire an instructor). The other challenge is finding a convenient place to skate. Of course, this depends to a large extent on where you live. Some cities have great places to skate, with paved paths in parks or by the beach. Another concern you may have is the cost: about $200 to $300 for beginner's Rollerblade skates, and another $100 to $200 for the helmet, protective gloves, knee and elbow pads, and wrist braces. Before making this investment, rent the equipment and arrange for private instruction. A good web site to check out is Rollerblade.com to get you started on prices and specifications of various types of equipment.

Water fitness

After I was hit by the car, I had to undergo extensive rehabilitation just to be able to walk again. My physical therapist decided that in light of my injuries, my rehab would be best done in the water. I know what you're thinking: no way am I putting on a bathing suit in public. I thought the same thing. I said to Jim, my physical therapist, "I don't want to wear a bathing suit." He replied, "Tawni, this isn't Baywatch. Get your butt in the water."

I trembled as I put on my suit. Sick to my stomach, I was physically grossed out by how I looked. I was bruised *and* fat. It was one of those moments when you have to reach pretty far down within yourself to hold your head up.

They wheeled me into the pool in a wheelchair (remember I couldn't walk). The most amazing thing happened. For the first time in my life, I weighed nothing. It's like I rediscovered water. Water has that marvelous buoyant effect that takes away your physical sensation of weight.

I began with range-of-motion exercises designed to allow me to do common tasks with my limbs. I was destined for four months of water fitness, but after only two weeks, I really felt I was making progress. My hips felt better, my shoulders didn't ache as much when I slept, and my joints didn't scream at me.

Now I'm hooked on water fitness. I work out at least a couple times a week on days when I am not running. Working out in water is fun and a great way to socialize with people. Most public pools, community centers,

mind body spirit

schools, and YMCAs have water fitness classes. They also have very supportive people who encourage each other to make a regular water workout worth it.

If you are not interested in cycling, maybe you want to make water fitness a regular part of your workout. Water fitness is a great aerobic workout and the big pluses include high resistance because of the water, and no impact on legs and feet like you get when running or walking.

Why water? Many people don't consider working out in water to be a serious workout. They think it's too easy, or that it isn't aerobic. Believe me, since water is at least 12 times more resistant than air, you have to work. That's why you feel like you're moving in slow motion in the water—*because* of the resistance. It is very much an aerobic workout, and it forces you to use all large muscles in your legs and arms.

The day after a long run, I want to move, but I don't want to stress my joints. That's why water is the perfect medium. Also, if you are injured like I was after my accident, if you struggle with ongoing exercise-related injuries like knee problems, or if you have a physical problem such as arthritis, water workouts are an ideal way to maintain your fitness level during recovery or to work out without putting strain on your joints.

Whenever I tell people I do water fitness once or twice a week, they look at me kind of funny and say, "Oh you mean swimming." Actually, I don't mean swimming. The water fitness I'm talking about is *vertical* water fitness that involves a flotation belt that keeps you (and your hair, thank God) above water. Your movement against the resistance of the water builds strength and improves your overall cardiovascular endurance. This is great for increasing your endurance for land-based exercises like walking, running, and cycling. It is also great for providing relief and improvement of joints as in my case with the osteoarthritis I developed after my accident.

A flotation belt is a special belt, usually made of a lightweight rubber foam material designed to be wrapped around your waist, enabling you to float in deep water up to your neck. The belt makes it possible for you to exercise your entire body without having to worry about sinking or remaining afloat. The belt also prevents you from bobbing up and down.

There are several manufacturers of these belts and the best ones that I am aware of are made by Aquajogger and Speedo. The cost is between $35 and $50. You can even increase resistance in the water by wearing special webbed gloves and water shoes also available from these companies. Check out the Aquajogger Web site at www.aquajogger.com for products and further information.

I recommend that if you want to give water fitness a try, check out your local public pool, YMCA, or local school for water fitness classes. If they offer classes, they probably provide the flotation belts and other gear. Of course, if you have your own pool you can purchase the belt and other gear. What's nice about going to a class is the support you get from your fellow water fitness classmates. It's a fun way to work out.

But what do you wear while working out in water? For one thing, avoid a suit manufactured of Lycra. Lycra does not wear well. Continuous exposure to chlorine will ultimately ruin a Lycra bathing suit.

Also rinse and line dry your suit after each time you use it. If you go to a public pool, take advantage of the swimsuit spinner they may have. If there is no spinner, you can keep your suit in a plastic bag until you take it home. But never wash your suit in a washing machine.

To keep from hurting the soles of your feet and to prevent athlete's foot, wear flip-flops, thongs, or rubber/plastic sandals to and from the pool, especially a public pool.

Water fitness expert, Juliana Larson, author of *Water Dance: Water Fitness For Mind, Body, & Soul,* observes that women are more inclined to work out in water than men. She even has a term to describe the process of women encouraging other women to workout in water. She calls the process *women*toring—women mentoring women. Women understand how embarrassed you may feel about how you look in a swimsuit, and they help you realize that it does not matter. Besides, when you are in the water, no one can see anything anyway. Women tend to be more nurturing to help you achieve your goals.

MY WATER FITNESS WORKOUT

I keep my workout pretty simple. I put on my flotation belt and enjoy running in the water, usually about 30 to 40 minutes, first up one end, and then back down to the other end of the pool. To keep this interesting, I try to at least vary my run by making one stretch a hard run, and the return stretch an easy run.

Now I have taken water fitness classes and even received personal water fitness instruction from water fitness expert Juliana Larson, in Eugene,

Oregon. Juliana taught me several very good water fitness workout routines that I want to share with you here as an alternative to just running in the pool from end to end.

Juliana has me start out with getting warmed up by doing range-of-motion movements, which is just another way to describe walking in the water while flexing, extending, and rotating all your joints (arms, hands, fingers, legs, feet, toes). From there we would do some jogging/running in place, followed by several water fitness routines.

One fun water fitness routine—that also happens to be a good work-out—is the Sit Kick. In deep water assume a sitting position, as if you are sitting in a chair. Your thighs don't move. You work your knees and ankles. As you sit, kick out toe up. Use a breaststroke motion or a paddlewheel motion with your arms to assist in the pull across the pool. Then extend your arms straight out to your sides—pull them in front of you and clap and take them to the back as best you can and clap. I try to repeat this maybe ten times.

Jumping rope

According to Covert Bailey, the fitness and diet expert who wrote the popular book, *Fit or Fat,* jumping rope is one of the most efficient ways to work out. It is both an upper and lower body workout, and gets your heart racing almost instantly. Another plus is that the equipment is cheap; you can purchase a jump rope for about ten dollars. The only problem is that it's not easy to do if you are very overweight, and I never did know how to work the rope very easily.

Many professional athletes like football players and boxers use rope jumping as a regular part of their workout routine. But those guys are already in fantastic shape and jumping rope is just a way to maintain their existing physical condition. I think jumping rope is okay, it's just not for me.

Video workouts and aerobics classes

Everyone knows about the popularity of Jane Fonda's aerobic workout videos. As I understand it, Jane made more money from the sales of her aerobic videos than the money she made from all her movies combined. But the question is: Do you know anyone who still uses the Jane Fonda workout videos? Probably not. Does that mean her tapes are not good? Not at all. Jane knows what she is talking about. The trouble is that videotapes are boring. Who wants to jump around in their living room in front of the tube every day for the rest of their lives to get fit? No one. At least, no one I know.

However, I do believe the one very good thing that came out of the popularity of Jane Fonda's videos is that it encouraged people to join aerobic exercise classes. And I definitely know people who do that practically every day. Plus videos are great for stay at home moms and can be a stepping stone for them as well.

An aerobics class can be fun, and it's a great way to stay motivated because you are sharing in the common goal of getting and staying fit. It is a very social experience. One of the reasons I like running races is that I get to spend time with Connectors. It is a wonderfully uplifting, motivating, inspiring social activity. Aerobic classes can serve this purpose, but aerobic videos rarely do this.

Strength training

Strength training is not aerobic exercise, but it is an important part of an overall fitness plan and a huge component of weight loss. Strength training, sometimes called weight training, involves lifting free weights or working out on a weight machine with various stations for upper and lower body workouts to build muscle strength. Why does this matter? For women it can help prevent debilitating diseases such as osteoporosis (deterioration of the bones). Generally, strength training tones muscles and is a nice blend with your cardiovascular workout; you feel stronger and look smaller. In addition, building your muscle tone can boost your metabolism.

MY ROUTINE FOR STRENGTH TRAINING

For my own routine, I like to include several very effective strengthening exercises. Now this does not mean that I want to add bulk—I don't want to look like a muscle man. I just want to get stronger to improve my overall running performance, and I want to develop lean muscular limbs. I usually strength train three times per week between running days. I often focus on my upper body to give my legs a rest on non-running days, but weight training should really be applied to your whole body. I call my strength-training work "Sleeveless in San Francisco" because it's my goal to develop great arms so I can wear a sleeveless outfit without being mortified. But I can see the definition in my legs, too, and that's a great reward!

So, on one of my strength training days I do exercises that emphasize my chest and shoulders. On another strength training day I emphasize my biceps

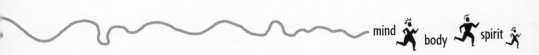

and triceps. Finally, I devote one strength training day to exercises for my back muscles. I usually do three or four sets of repetitions for each exercise.

I won't suggest a particular weight for these exercises. That is something that varies from person to person. If you've never done weight training before, then definitely get instructions and a step-by-step beginner's program from the weight trainer at the gym. The weight trainer will be able to assess your strength and fitness level and design a progressive program that you can follow without injuring yourself. Obviously, some people are naturally stronger. The amount of weight you start with should push you, but not too hard. You don't want to strain or injure yourself, so take it easy. Over time, as you maintain a regular strength-training routine, you will get stronger and you will know when to increase weight to make your workout more challenging. But it's a good idea to check in with the weight trainer before you make any major adjustments to your routine or the amount of weight you're using.

Even though I don't work my legs in the gym because I'm giving them a rest from running, there are a number of good weight exercises you can do to build muscle strength, endurance, and tone in your upper and lower legs. You'll also want to incorporate exercises for your chest and shoulders, for your upper arms (triceps) and lower arms (biceps), and for your back. Plenty of good books on basic weight training exercises are available, and the gym's trainer is also there to help you develop an overall program.

Old-fashioned exercises

Two exercises that you used to do in PE class when you were a kid—push-ups and sit-ups—are good complements to a fitness routine and help build strength.

I do push-ups as a way to strengthen my back and arms. Now, I have to do the wimpy push-ups with my knees on the floor because otherwise I couldn't do more than two or three! If you're going to do push-ups on the floor, you can keep your knees and calves on the ground and just push up your torso with your arms.

If you don't want to do push-ups on the floor, you can compromise by finding a stable desk or table and lean against that with your arms. You can then lower and raise your whole body and the strain is more evenly distributed; this enables you to adjust the angle and increase the intensity of the lifting as you get stronger.

Sit-ups are a good way to strengthen your abdominal muscles. I can hear you groaning, but there are easy and effective ways to do sit-ups. One way I like to do them is to lie on the floor (preferably carpeted if you value your back and butt) or on an exercise pad. Put your feet up on a chair or on one of those giant exercise balls. Place your hands behind your head and point your elbows straight out to either side. When you lift, concentrate on lifting with your stomach muscles and keeping your back flat on the ground. To remind myself of that, I use my chin as an arrow to point toward the ceiling and make sure I'm where I am supposed to be during the sit-ups.

You don't have to come all the way up to your legs. Coming up to the point where you feel a strain is good. You can add to the intensity of the sit-up by not allowing your shoulder blades to touch the ground behind you as you are doing a set of ten or whatever you can do that day.

Fitness equipment

We should talk a little about exercise equipment here. There are many products out there. And naturally, every manufacturer wants you to believe their product offers the best way to achieve the best aerobic workout. I'll tell you my experience with various types of equipment. Right now, I want you to know that I don't think it is absolutely necessary to spend a huge amount of money on exercise equipment at the outset. But obviously, in the end, you decide what is best for you and your circumstances.

Should you decide to go with a piece of exercise equipment of any kind, remember the best kind to buy is the one you'll really use. It's like clothes. You don't just buy clothes because they're on sale and you don't just buy exercise equipment unless you're making a realistic decision for you, not for someone else's intentions. This is both a lifestyle change and a sizable financial commitment.

The only way to know what equipment you are likely to use is to get out there and start looking at some. Test different types at a local gym or a friendly equipment store. Don't be daunted. Just tell the salesperson, "Hey, I'm just starting out. What can work for me?" That way you'll learn your options. You don't *have* to buy the first piece of equipment you look at either. Before you buy anything, you may also want to check out articles in consumer or fitness magazines, like *Consumer Reports,* that rank the latest in exercise equipment.

mind body spirit

Two things will guide you in the equipment realm. Ideally, the equipment you buy will work your whole body or major areas of it. That way you'll be likely to burn more calories. Secondly, the more you use your equipment, the more calories you'll burn. My treadmill wasn't burning much when I was using it as a clothes hangar!

Treadmills

Speaking of treadmills. I started getting serious about my fitness by getting on a treadmill. A treadmill can be a good way of beating those "excuses blues," of defeating the mindset that it's too cold, hot, rainy, snowy, whatever. Treadmills worked for me when I was traveling for my job and I didn't want to run in a strange city, especially as early as I got up in the mornings.

Recently, while running with Oprah during a Susan Komen Breast Cancer awareness 5K (3.1 miles) race (in which only women can participate) in October last year, Oprah mentioned to me that in recent months she had been doing most of her running on a treadmill. She indicated something that I too noticed: It ain't like running outside. For some reason, it just does not seem like you get as good a workout. Of course, this may be more of a mental thing, and less a physical thing. Because, remember, ultimately the goal is to get your heart rate up enough, long enough to make it aerobic and to make it burn fat. And there is no question that a treadmill can help you get your heart rate up.

A recent study in the IJO of more than 5,000 men and women between 40 and 60 showed that perseverance really does pay off. Each one-minute improvement in treadmill time reduces the chance of an 11-pound weight gain by 14% in men and by 9% in men, and the chance of a 22-pound gain by 21% in both men and women. Definitely a good argument for baby steps!

INTERNATIONAL JOURNAL OF OBESITY, VOL. 23, ISSUE 3, PP. 320-327

One thing I learned about treadmills is that you definitely get what you pay for. Generally, if you get a treadmill for less than $1,500, you will probably not be able to run on it. Vigorous walking is the limit; otherwise you ruin the machine. To be able to run, you need a heavy duty, well-built treadmill especially designed to withstand running. These start at about $2,000. But then you also get all sorts of useful features like calories burned calculation, speed, distance, and a timing program, along with incline adjustments and other features.

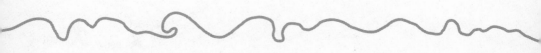

Runner's World regularly rates treadmills and that's a good place to start before you step out the door to buy. You can find their ratings at www.runnersworld.com.

Stationary cycles

I also like the idea of a stationary bike. Again, it's one of those pieces of equipment that can be a standby when you're having a lazy day or weather from hell. It's also excellent for cross-training because it works your muscles in a different way than when you're walking or running. If you've injured yourself, using a stationary bike can help you maintain your fitness level without aggravating your injury.

Cross-country machines

One of the most popular and widely known machines designed to simulate cross-country snow skiing is the NordicTrack. The thing about this type of workout is that it is a highly intensive aerobic workout. I mean this thing really works. The trouble is that it is tricky to learn how to use it, hard to find a place to store it, and it is expensive—the introductory machine starts at just under $1,000. Of course, some people prefer the actual activity outdoors using real skis on real snow.

Stair-steppers

These machines are a fairly good workout and fairly easy to do, but the emphasis is on the lower body. The other thing is that these machines come in all types of shapes and styles. Most of the cheap variety consist of piston technology. These are junk and will not last long. The best stair stepper is the Stairmaster. But you need to be prepared to spend the big bucks on this apparatus, way past $2,000. I personally would rather spend my money (much less) and time on a stationary bike.

Rowing machines

To me, these seem like a weird way to work out. But these machines that simulate rowing a boat are actually a pretty good way to get aerobic. Most people don't realize that a good rowing machine forces you to use your upper body *and* your lower body to do the workout properly. But the emphasis is your upper body; for me this fact alone is a reason not to use it. Also, as with the stair stepping machine, a good rowing machine is an expensive piece of equipment. And when travelling, which I do a lot, you are not going to easily find a rowing machine, not even at a gym.

mind · body · spirit

Weight/strength training equipment

I belong to a gym, so that's where I do my weight work, and I feel that that works for me. At some point in the future, I may want to invest in a home gym, if only for the timesaving factor. A home gym would ideally have upper and lower body workout stations. In other words, I would be able to exercise my legs (quads, glutes, and adductor/abductor muscles) and my arms (biceps, triceps, shoulders, etc.). A good, basic system that works these muscles starts at about $1,000.

REST BETWEEN WORKOUTS

If you're like me, once you catch the health and fitness bug, you might tend to be compulsive and want to exercise every single day. But realize that what you are doing by working your muscles is actually tearing down and then subsequently building up strength and endurance. Therefore, your body *needs* a day of rest between working out, especially when you start out.

You need to condition your body to accept the changes that are happening. If you force things to go forward too quickly you could get injured. And an injury can be very challenging to get past. I'll talk more about that in the next chapter, but for now, I encourage you to schedule at least one day of rest per week into your fitness routine, and an additional day if you have just done a particularly difficult workout.

WHEN NOT TO WORK OUT

I don't advise that you go out in the middle of 90-plus degrees and exercise. I remember when the comedian Martin Lawrence went running in Los Angeles in 105 degrees; he collapsed and went into a coma. The same goes for extreme cold weather. I know that in some places winter is so cold that you have to breathe through a scarf to avoid damaging your lungs. Besides, there are other hazards to running or walking on snow or ice, like slipping and falling on your behind.

So use common sense and if the weather is at extremes, exercise inside on a treadmill or a piece of stationary exercise equipment.

Cross-training

Why cross-training? In other words, why engage in an additional aerobic exercise when you've already found one that works? For example, I found running, but I also cross-train with water fitness and cycling. Why not just keep running and not do any other aerobic exercise?

I agree with most of the experts who say you should do one thing and do it well. But I also like to put a little variety into my workout, if only for boredom's sake. It's good for a number of other reasons, too.

Cross-train for recovery/rest

After you race or have a long run, it's a good idea to either take a day off, but if you want to do *something*, water fitness or a stationary bike are good ways of giving your legs a breather. While you do get in an aerobic workout, you aren't pushing yourself the way you would by running. I don't view cross-training as a *replacement* for running, but if you have just run a marathon and would like a few weeks off without turning into a total couch potato, cross-training is something you can do three to five times a week. That way when you do run again, it's not like you have never run in your life. Every so often, a break can help your motivation level, too.

Cross-train during lousy weather

Yep, we all have days like these! You open your eyes and the first thing you see is rain slapping against the window or snow flakes drifting down silently. Or worse, there's been an ice storm overnight and there's literally no way of running or walking outside without ending up on your butt. These are all good reasons for an alternative workout source, like a tread-mill, stationary bike, or stair stepper.

This doesn't mean you never go walking or running in the rain; that's what Gore-tex and Activent fabrics are for. But again, this is reality. Some-times not even the most technologically advanced clothing can force you out the door.

Having some cross-training equipment inside will assure that you feel "fitness chipper" even when the weather outside is gloomy.

Cross-train when injured

This is two-fold. Not only can you rest your injuries while cross-training, but you can cross-train to help prevent them as well. For example, running can be jarring to your whole body at times. When you are sore or become injured and cannot run, cross-training can help fight off that panicked feel-ing of "Oh my God, I'm not running and now I'm going to get fat!"

Plus, done properly, cross-training is aerobic and can give overall strength to muscles not directly used in running or walking, thus making you stronger and less injury-prone. Overall, cross-training keeps you fit and

mind body spirit

Awareness and attitude are the two biggest factors in keeping yourself safe as a woman walker or runner. While we would like to believe that nothing will ever happen to us, the facts fly in the face of such reasoning. We have had the statistics drummed into us for years, but more important than just remembering facts is adjusting our thinking patterns. Yes, you can affirm yourself as a powerful woman, a self-confident being who is out there getting in shape, mentally and physically. I would only add that you check that with some basic common sense.

- Don't run scared, but *do* run **aware.** Your awareness may include a plan of action you developed by taking a self-defense class. Save the headphones for the treadmill. You cannot be as aware as you need to be when you are distracted by music.

- Running or walking with a **self-defense spray** visible to others may act to deter possible attacks, but also has the benefit of making you feel better mentally—tougher even.

- By virtue of running in technologically advanced fabrics that tend to be both lighter and more scant, some people might say that women invite trouble. I would argue that it's not what you're wearing, it's how you're wearing it. **Look people in the eye** like the defiant woman warrior that you are when you run by and you help place yourself outside the category of women likely to be attacked.

- A **morning workout** versus an evening one *can* be more safe, just in terms of there being more light. However, I strongly suggest that you are aware of the neighborhood that you are running in and your surroundings—people and environment—in general. If there's any doubt in your mind that you won't be any safer in the morning than in the evening, go to a club to work out, work out with a friend, or work out in your home with a treadmill you purchase.

- **Always listen to your instincts.** Don't push away that inner voice; it's trying to keep you *alive.*

- In the case of safety, you are allowed to be what would otherwise be considered rude. Someone stopping to "ask directions," etc. can be met with a firm "no" and you don't have to feel guilty about it. **You don't have to engage in conversation,** especially if someone makes you uncomfortable. Don't believe that you can rationalize with someone either. Just keep moving.

- If there's any question about the area you run or walk in, **arrange to meet another person** there to work out. Stay in your car until he or she arrives or, better yet, meet at a designated safe place and go from there.

makes you perform better in your first choice activity. In my case, that would be running.

Your fitness routine summary

Before you embark on a regular fitness routine, it is important to keep several important elements in focus. I'll list the five most important things for you to be aware of:

1 **Choose one main workout activity for your routine.** Make sure that activity is aerobic and something you know you can do consistently, most likely for the rest of your life.

2 **Decide on all aspects of your routine.** Work into your plan exercises for stretching, flexibility, strengthening, and endurance.

3 **Understand the advantages of cross-training.** Try various cross-training activities and then choose one or two to add to your fitness plan.

4 **Always plan a day of rest or an easy workout day in your routine.** A day of rest isn't a cop-out; it's an important part of your plan to help prevent injury.

5 **Whatever you do during your routine, always make sure you engage in an activity that is safe in all respects.** Pay attention to location, time of day, how you engage in that activity, and proper coaching.

mind   body   spirit

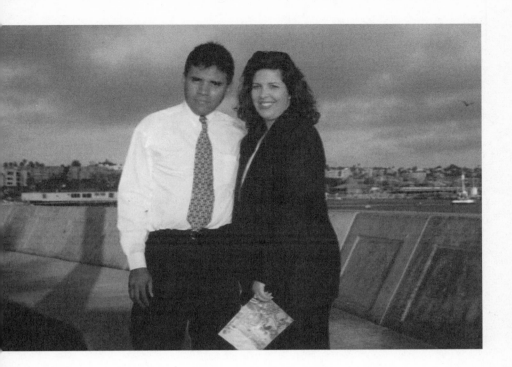

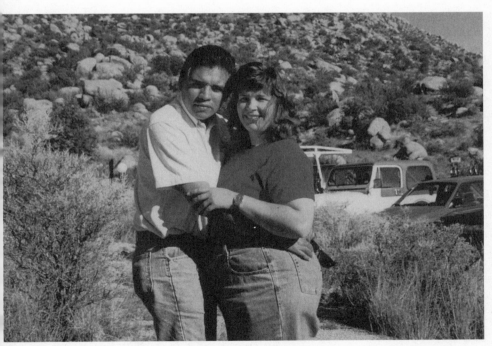

July '96, Martin and I at the ocean and the desert. I'm 225 pounds in these photos

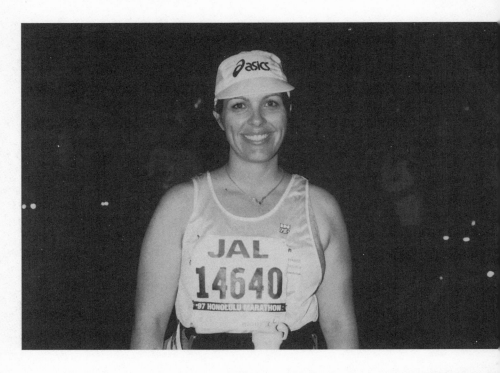

Me at my first marathon, the '97
Honolulu Marathon

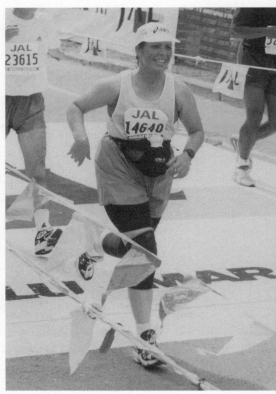

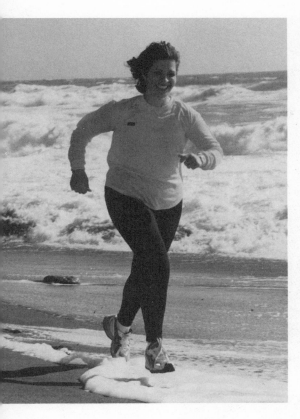

Here I am running at my favorite place, the beach near my home in San Francisco

Me with San Francisco Connectors, Debbie (left) and Martha, Nov. '97

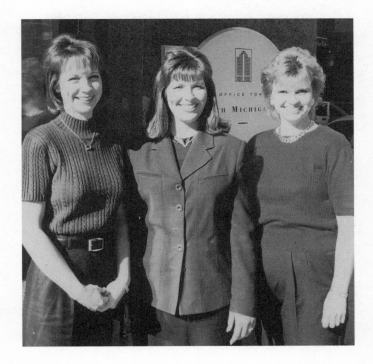

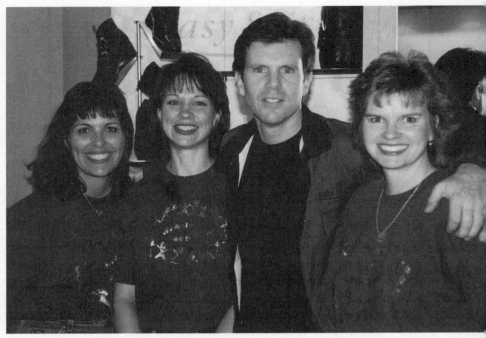

Debbie, Martha and I meet Bob Greene for the first time, Nov. '97

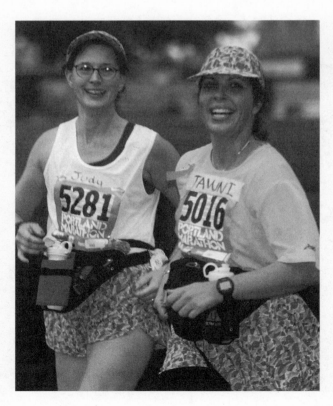

Me with New Jersey Connector, Judy, running together at the '98 Portland, OR Marathon

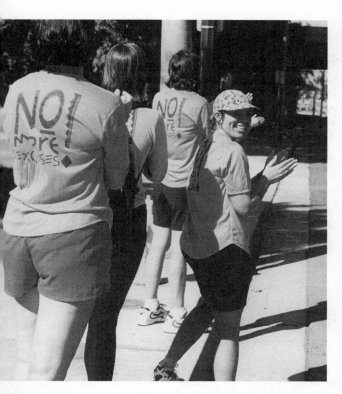

Me with San Jose Connectors at the '99 Silicon Valley Marathon

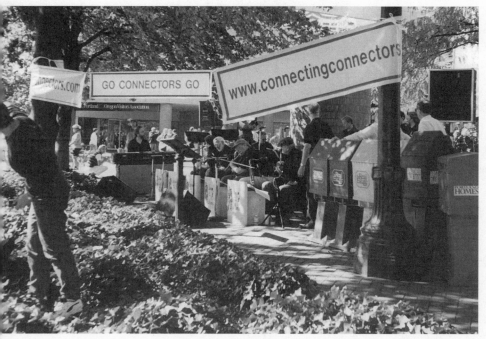

The connectingconnectors.com banner proudly displayed at the '99 Portland, OR Marathon

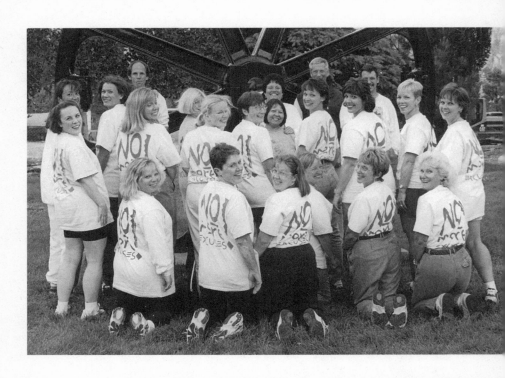

Me with Eugene, OR Connectors at Jeff Galloway's training workshop

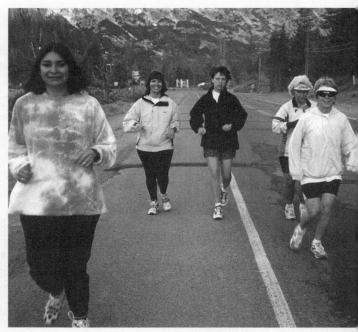

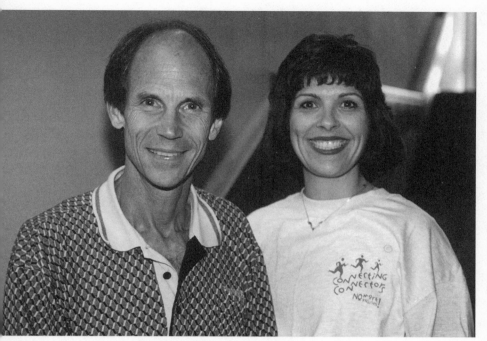

eff Galloway, veteran marathoner and author, April '99

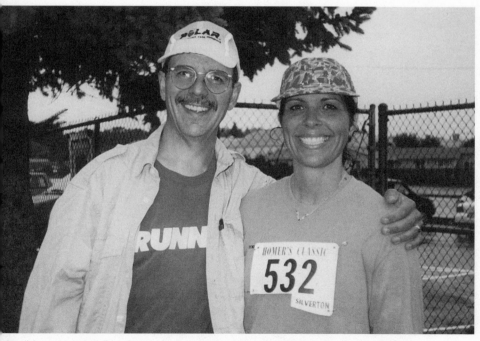

ohn "the penguin" Bingham, distance runner, bestselling author, August '99

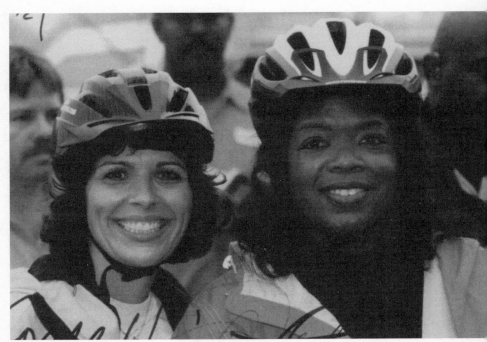

Oprah and I just before we began Bob Greene's bicycle trek across America, April '99

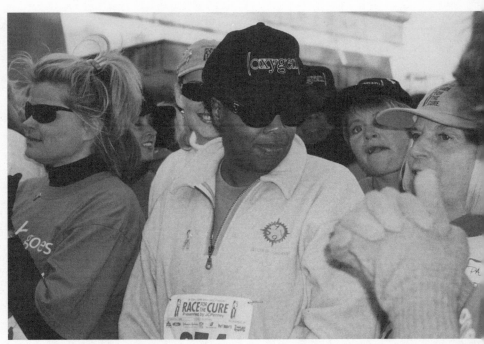

I ran with Oprah at the Race For The Cure (breast cancer benefit), Madison, Wisconsin, Oct'99

Fitness challenges

It's been two months since I pulled my hamstring/butt muscle in the San Jose Mercury News 10K. I'm so depressed I can't run. I keep trying and it still hurts. I'm scared to death I'm going to gain all my weight back. I know better than to think this way, but I can't help it.

I've tried massage, acupuncture, the chiropractor, jacuzzi, ice, you name it I've tried it. I've rested it. What more can I do but wait? I hate this.

I haven't lost a single POUND this year and it's already MAY! I swore I would be at Goal weight by the time I run the Portland Marathon in October. And with the way things are looking I'll be lucky if I don't gain. God this is frustrating. How can it be possible to workout 5-6 days a week, watch what I eat and still NOT LOSE A SINGLE POUND! Not fair. I often wonder why the hell I even try.

People think it's easy for me because I've lost a lot of weight already, but let me tell you I get frustrated almost every month when I see I have "only lost a pound." I can train for a marathon and still "only lose 1-2 pounds a month." NOT FAIR.

Now that I can't run I'm terrified I'm going to gain weight. I'm doing my best to cross train by swimming and biking but it's not the same. I feel really depressed. I feel like I don't have much to share with my group because I'm not out exercising. I have signed up for all these races and now I can't do them because of this damn injury. NOT FAIR.

JOURNAL ENTRY, MAY 11, 1998

L ike it or not, no matter how careful you are, no matter how gradually you increase your exercise time and push your physical limits to condition your body for greater performance, invariably you get injured. Added to that there seems to be the tendency to sacrifice your workouts in the name of work, stress, illness, or other chaos that makes its way into your life. All these things pose a challenge to your regular fitness routine and sometimes make you want to give up. You just want to throw your hands up and shout: "What's the use?!"

But don't give up! Hang in there. Oftentimes, just keeping on is enough to make the difference in your life. It's just what you need to do.

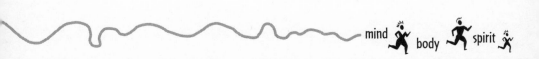

mind   body   spirit

Stress

Exercise and working out are the best things you can do for yourself during times of stress, but typically they are the first things thrown out when you perceive that you need more time for yourself. Ironically, the exercise *is* for you; you just need a major change in perspective. When your health is on the top of your priority list, there's no question of it being thrown out in times of chaos. During this time, go over your goals. If you need to write them down again to remind yourself of their importance, now's the time. You had the drive and determination to put them down in the first place, so don't let that slip away.

I decided to try running to help me deal with stress and a horrible sleeping prob-
lem. All the stress in my life had turned me into quite the insomniac. I eventually
made it to two miles and stayed at that distance for several months. Now since
my involvement with the Connectors, I have run a 1/2 marathon, a 20K, and
plan to run my first marathon in October. I am sleeping better; I have energy to
spare; and, I have a wonderful support system in place.   MELODY, CONNECTING IN FL

Mental challenges

Sometimes no matter how focused you are, you have days when you cannot get yourself to exercise. Or you need to get back on the exercise wagon after you have fallen off due to a break or sickness, injury or plain laziness. Here are some things you can reflect on:

1 It is important to just tell yourself that there really is no starting and stopping. It's much harder to get 'back on track' than to just stick with it. Where you are now will pass, and as you continue, what challenged you today, will mean nothing in the weeks, months, and years ahead. Simply do not allow a passing moment to disrupt a lifelong commitment. It is not an option.

2 Sometimes you may have to evaluate more closely why you 'got off track' in the first place? If your answer is because it was the holidays, or it was summer or (pick one), then you might have the "diet mentality."

The fact is I remind myself at these challenging moments that I really have worked (I've been at this for 3 years) at changing the way I look at exercise and eating healthy. I am not on a diet so there is no starting and stopping. If I miss a day or two of exercise, so what, no big deal. If I eat poorly one day or at one meal, so what. This is a lifetime thing.

3 Okay, so you've officially fallen off the wagon and you want back on: great! The first step is missing what you once had. So, my advice is *start*. Don't blame yourself and start coming up with excuses. Just start again. What is done is done. Yesterday is gone; tomorrow is a new day, and the beginning of a new life.

Lay out your clothes the night before, set your alarm, wake up, put your shoes on and go. Get rid of the yucky food (you know, the fats, the sugars, all that tempting stuff) in your house and replace it with healthy food. Start drinking your water and drink some more when you don't feel like it. Commit to one step and just concentrate on doing one thing. Do just one small thing for a full 24 hours and then start concerning yourself with the next thing the next 24 hours. Start small and build on your first day's success. Being good to your body for 24 to 48 hours will do wonders for you mentally.

4 Learn from your experience. What could you have done differently? Proper planning can be a real lifesaver. If the yucky food isn't in the house, it's pretty hard to eat it. If you plan on meeting somebody to work out, you'll get yourself there 90 percent of the time. If you don't have anyone to meet, then log on and commit to the group and be accountable. It works just as well. Honest!

5 Next time your schedule gets out of whack, stop for a moment. Take a deep breath and remind yourself of *what* you want and *how* you want to feel in your body. Reflect on why you started your fitness and health program in the first place. Sometimes just a small mental nudge can be all it takes to get back on track.

Physical challenges

Embarking on your new fitness journey will bring you a lot closer to your body. I know it sounds silly—how could we *be* any closer to our bodies, right? But you will learn to *listen* to your body and take your action cues from what it tells you.

Normal aches & pains vs. injuring yourself

You may experience two different kinds of discomfort while working out. The first one will feel like an ache, perhaps in some area of your body

mind body spirit

that is being newly exercised. You will feel a dull, resonant discomfort. This isn't bad! Actually, it's pretty normal. Say that you feel it in your quadriceps (upper leg muscles). You can either just ignore these aches or you can take something like Advil, aspirin, or some similar pain reliever.

A recent study of 40,000 female nurses aged 46-71 revealed that a weight gain of between five and 20 pounds had a significant effect on their daily activities. Things that we think nothing of—dressing, bathing, walking up stairs, bending, carrying objects, etc.—become difficult. The study also asserted that overweight women who lost even a small amount of weight had an easier time with daily functions.

JOURNAL OF AMERICAN MEDICAL ASSOCIATION (JAMA), DECEMBER 8, 1999

The second kind of discomfort is a sharp pain that feels like a stab in a muscle or tendon area. You may not be able to put weight on your leg or to use the affected muscle. This is definitely your body telling you to ease up. An ice compress on the tender area and just staying off your feet can address this type of challenge.

Just be aware that when you first start exercising, you need to learn to be in tune with your body. Listen to what it is telling you and be reasonable. Overexerting will only end up discouraging you and physically damaging to your body in the long run.

As I indicated a moment ago, the nice thing is that you *will* become more in tune with your body as you continue your fitness routine. You will learn through experience when a certain ache or pain is something to be concerned about. You will also learn when to take a break for recovery, and when it's okay to keep going. It's amazing to me how disconnected with my body I had been all my life. This may seem strange, but unless you exercise, you probably are not really very in tune with your body.

Blisters

When you start walking or running long distances, sooner or later you will find little blisters cropping up here and there on your feet. It seems so strange to me when I hear people complain that walking or running causes blisters and that they would rather not walk or run than get blisters. What's the big deal? Maybe it's because they don't understand what a blister is and think of it as a bad thing to get blisters. I mean it's not like your foot is going to drop off or something. Anyway, here is a simple explanation of a blister: a blister is formed when there is friction against your skin, causing fluid to form beneath the skin and a raised area that is the blister.

How do blisters come about? You can get blisters if your shoes don't fit properly. Perhaps the shoe is too tight across the toes and you get a blister on the side of your big toe. If you're a beginning runner, you may get blisters in the course of conditioning your feet to get used to running.

Now that you have the blister, how do you get rid of it? Basically the same way that you prevent them. Keep your feet dry. Make sure that you have a proper fit in your shoes and that your current pair hasn't gotten so old and are worn in areas (if so, replace them). You can also alternate between thin socks and slightly thicker, padded socks that can protect your heel and toe areas.

My favorite way to prevent blisters is greasing my toes and any other place I might have rubbing with Body Glide, the most magical product in the world. I have prevented more blisters and chafing with Body Glide than with anything else I have tried, including Vaseline (which doesn't work).

Side aches

Side aches are most often caused by not breathing correctly or not breathing enough. If you feel a side ache coming on, you can try several things. Try what I call "tall breathing." You can even do this without stopping. Stand up straight and breathe in and out deeply, in effect, "stretching" your diaphragm and allowing more air in. You can even throw your arms over your head as you do this to stretch your diaphragm to the fullest.

Another way to zap a side ache is to change the way you breathe. Pay attention to the way you are breathing at the time you start getting a side ache and then try breathing in more deeply and blowing air out more forcefully. A change as small as that can often derail a potentially painful cramp.

Side aches can also be a sign that you are not breathing enough for the pace you are running or walking or cycling or whatever. Either increase your breathing or slow down the pace of your exercise and you will probably get rid of the cramp.

If I get a side ache as I am running and none of the above methods work, I even poke a few fingers into where it is aching. Massaging around or poking slightly into the cramped area while continuing to breathe in and out deeply can alleviate the side ache.

Sickness

We've all had it happen. You wake up in the morning, feverish, a stuffy nose, and a sore throat. Maybe you can still force yourself to go running,

mind body spirit

but a few days go by and your cold is in full swing. No way do you feel like exercising, but is it right *not* to? The fact is that your body really does need rest like doctors tell you when you are sick. The reason is that your body actually needs the protein that you burn off in a workout to repair itself during an illness. So besides the fact that you don't feel like working out, you are probably better off not straining your body during an illness.

Try not to let a period of illness frustrate you. Don't think:"Oh no! I can already feel my fat cells expand at the very thought of sitting around being sick." Just remember: you have already made the commitment that you are going to be fit and healthy for life. Just because you are sick now, does not mean that you are not going to continue to maintain your fitness routine. You are. Being sick is just part of life. So hang in there; this too shall pass.

Common injuries

Generally, the injuries you get from running or walking can be combated with using ice, anti-inflammatory medicine (like Advil, Tylenol or some ibuprofen-based pain reliever) and resting (i.e., not exerting the injured area). In addition, I find that stretching is usually the most effective method of preventing injuries, particularly injuries that could result from strained muscles and tendons. So you can recognize common injuries, I'll outline some of what can happen when you do run or walk consistently.

Achilles tendon

Tendons are what connect your muscles to your bones. Many times you can get an inflammation as the result of overexertion in a particular tendon that is in your calf muscle where it attaches to the heel bone. You'll feel pain near the heel in the back of your leg, enough so that you may be reluctant to run or walk. You have gotten Achilles tendonitis because your calf muscles or Achilles tendons were not properly stretched and conditioned to endure a lot of uphill running or simply a sudden increase in your overall running distance.

What do you do to recover and get back out there ASAP? In this case, definitely listen to your body and stay off you feet for a while! If I feel pain in my Achilles, I apply ice packs (frozen peas still packed in the plastic package also work well) every three or four hours for 20 minutes each time. You may also be able to alleviate the pain by elevating your leg(s). The idea here is to treat this problem immediately, not to try and run through it. You can cause more problems doing that and lose much more of your ability to work out by not addressing the pain right away.

The speed at which you recover from an Achilles injury depends on the shape you are in, but generally you can return to your activity when you cannot feel pain in your Achilles when walking or running. Also, you should be able to put weight on the leg without discomfort and you can jump up or ascend stairs without noticing any pain. Be patient; recovery could take up to six weeks, and that can be frustrating. I suggest engaging in a non-impact aerobic activity like outdoor or stationary cycling or water fitness during this period. If you are concerned about maintaining strength in your legs during this period, you may also include leg strength training exercises using a strength training machine.

Preventing Achilles injuries starts with stretching your calf muscles and Achilles tendons prior to running or walking (or whatever exercise you do).

Just to let you know, there are many scary stories about people who ignore an Achilles injury and this results in a rupture of the tendon. This literally means the tendon snaps in two. Usually when this happens there is a distinct popping sound like someone firing a gun, and you cannot walk on your leg. They repair extreme (and fairly unusual) cases like this surgically to reattach the tendon. For years various athletes, particularly football players, have tended to suffer Achilles tendon ruptures because of the constant stress on these ligaments during such a rough and tumble sport. But in nearly every case, such injuries can be avoided, and stretching is an important way to safeguard against Achilles problems.

Hamstring

You have probably heard baseball players or other runners talk about hamstring injuries. That is because they are pretty common. Your hamstrings are muscles that run along the back of your thighs and are what you use to pull your thighs backward and bend your knees. That's simplifying it some since your hamstrings are pretty central to any kind of exercise you do.

When you feel hamstring pain, rest, ice and elevation are in order, as well as mild drugs like Advil or other ibuprofen brand. However, a hamstring injury can be serious enough that you may want to consult a physician or sports medicine specialist. Regular stretching is a major way of preventing a hamstring injury as is strength training your legs with weight work.

mind body spirit

Runner's knee

I could call it by its scientific name, but most runners know it as runner's knee, so that's what I'll stick with. You get it as a result of the persistent pounding your ligaments and muscles around your kneecap endure while you are running and to a lesser extent while walking. Again, as a beginning runner especially, you have not been conditioned enough to endure the pounding and strain on your kneecaps because of running. For many people, runner's knee can be very painful as a nagging, throbbing pain, even when you're not running. At the very least you may feel uncomfortable walking or running, especially down hills or stairs, and you may even have swelling in the knee area or hear popping when you put weight on it.

All these sound like great reasons not to run, don't they?! And I am aware that many people cite this type of pain as the reason they do not run. They view it as something you cannot overcome. The ironic part is that the more you run, the more you develop the muscles (quads) and ligaments in that area which actually "protect" the kneecap from receiving the pressure of your workout. I have heard mixed advice about dealing with runner's knee. Some say you should not run, or at least try to condition yourself gradually. Others say that you should run like normal to facilitate the conditioning process. You often hear: *"You need to run through it."*

I do know that once your knees have been conditioned, that eventually the pain will dissipate. Meanwhile, as you continue to run despite the discomfort, you can treat the knee with ice, similar to the way you treat an Achilles injury. You can also take Advil or some ibuprofen-based painkiller just before you run, and after you ran. As far as prevention is concerned, besides conditioning, properly supportive shoes can play a large part in preventing or at least reducing the discomfort of runner's knee. Of course, oddly enough, there are those people who never seem to be affected by runner's knee.

Aching shoulder & back aches

Sometimes I'm running along happily and I suddenly get this gnawing, aching feeling in one or the other shoulder. The first few times I didn't know what was happening but I have since learned that this is a sign of muscle fatigue: the result of keeping my arm tense.

The only way to overcome this is to first be aware that you are too tense, and then make a concerted effort to pay attention to your performance. If you tend to get tense, force yourself to keep your arm moving like your other arm with a 90-degree swing. Don't hold it straight or stiffen your arm. To overcome any immediate stiffness or aching, you may also want to roll your arm like winding it up for a pitch, like baseball pitchers do. Just swing it around real big several times and keep it moving. You should feel some relief when you do this from time to time.

Sometimes you may experience a backache just as you begin your exercise, or as you are already well into it. Believe it or not, this is because of poor posture. You may unconsciously be hunching over or slouching as you run. Work on keeping your head up, chin straight, shoulders aligned with hips, and chest out while running or walking, particularly long distances.

Shin splints

If you feel pain on the front of your lower leg below your knee and above your ankle, you may have a case of shin splints. You'll feel discomfort over your shinbone or in the muscles on either side of your shin. You'll get this from overuse, from increasing your mileage suddenly or by changing the surface you walk or run on. In addition, if you naturally tend to over-pronate (your foot flattens out more than normal), you can also have the tendency toward shin splints. You may have pain while you're resting or while you exercise (or both).

Icing your legs after each run with compresses, a cold wash cloth or even frozen peas can help reduce the chance of inflammation and may prevent shin splints. Since shin splints are another overuse injury, you can get ahead of the game by exercising gradually just like with runner's knee. This is another one of the "running through it" quirks of running. Also, make sure your shoes have the proper support and are not worn out.

Another critical thing to be aware of is the surface that you run on. Don't run on concrete, like sidewalks, even though you may think it's safer to do so. Sure, maybe for brief distances, but always try to run on asphalt, gravel, grass or anything other than concrete. If you are a beginner, you may not realize how hard concrete is on your feet and legs. An asphalt street is "softer" than concrete, because asphalt has more "give." As a distance runner, you'll want to run on the street no matter what.

mind body spirit

Finally, to avoid shin splints, and most other injuries for that matter, make sure you warm up and stretch before and after working out. Don't be stubborn about this! Taking the time to warm up will save you repeated injuries later.

Stress fractures

Usually stress fractures occur when you have been doing some form of repetitive activity and most often too much too soon. Stress fractures need to be diagnosed by bone scan and a "hot spot" being present or by an X-ray (however, with the latter method the stress fracture must be healing and calcium must be deposited in the region of the stress fracture for it to show up). Most commonly you will find that stress fractures will hurt with any and all activity whereas shin splints will hurt with only certain activities (Example: running long distances).

Allow your stress fractures to heal by taking a break from your regular activity and engaging in a different, non-impact activity like water fitness or cycling until the injury has healed. As with Achilles injuries, it is best to stay off your feet perhaps up to six weeks. Again, added to the non-impact activity, you can do some leg strength training to your recovery routine.

I get up at 5:45 am every day to workout because it is the one hour of the day that is 100 percent mine, and each day I choose to enjoy it by working out. Keeping my heart in shape and keeping my spirit in shape are the real needs being met by my morning workout.   MARY BETH, CONNECTING IN IL

The keys to fitness challenges

There are five key things you should know when faced with fitness challenges which are the result of an injury, or various aches and pains that prevent you from working out:

1 **Believe that you will get through whatever challenges you.** When I was laying in that hospital bed, feeling the frustration over not being able to do anything about the fact that someone had hit me with their car, I still knew that I would not go back to the way I was before. I knew that I was not going to allow this circumstance to make me feel sorry for myself. I knew I would get through this, and continue, not losing my focus. And I did and I am stronger today because I went through it.

2 **Treat your physical injury, ache, or pain, illness, by some physical means** (e.g., resting, taking Advil, using ice, etc.) **or see a physician.**

3 **Try alternate non-impact workouts, if appropriate.** Obviously this would not apply if you have the flu, or some other illness. In such cases you need to bide your time and let your body do its job of healing you.

4 **Make good food choices.** You already know what you should or should not eat. When you have to cut down or stop exercising for a period, just realize that you just have to continue doing what you have been doing all along. Don't worry about suddenly getting fat. Remember: your body still needs food, and starving yourself only forces your body to go into starvation mode, which means instead of using your fat stores, it saves them. Food is fuel so just make the best food choices. Also, don't forget to drink lots of water.

CHAPTER 7

Training for life

I'm still in SHOCK that I'm training for my first marathon. I notice over and over again how marathon training is a metaphor for life. It's really forcing me to keep my priorities straight. Since my long training walk is on Sunday, I'm getting to bed early on Saturday night. I'm making better food choices all week because I don't want to have an upset stomach for my long training walk on Sunday. It's a metaphor for life because life is a marathon, not a sprint. It's about taking life one day at a time, just as in a marathon you take it mile by mile, sometimes step by step. Training encompasses all aspects of my life. I see how everything is connected. It's been a long time since I've been proud of myself and my efforts and I think I'm finally beginning to see the importance of making myself a priority.

JOURNAL ENTRY, OCTOBER 25, 1997

I call this chapter "training for life" because I want to emphasize that being healthy and fit translates into being able to do much more than just run races or marathons. It means that you will be able to do things that you might never have thought you could. Your training and workouts can extend to all facets of your life and indeed as you get fit and make healthy food choices, you will be surprised at all the things you can do!

The way I can keep my training for life in perspective is to continuously give myself goals. Oftentimes I give myself just a series of little goals that add up to one big goal. Sometimes these goals are hour to hour—I must drink another glass of water before 3 pm, I just have to make it around that corner at the stop sign and then I'm half way done, etc.

A goal reached

I love to participate in races because they give me a goal to train for. I am also very competitive. Of course, I don't expect to actually win any of the races I enter. I mean, what normal person can run a mile in 6 minutes or less? I am competing with myself in a sense. I have given myself the goal to finish a race as quickly as I can.

Maybe you think you're not competitive. I used to think that, too. What I find interesting is that I have seen people who firmly insist that they are

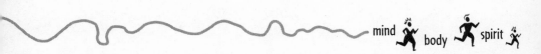

mind　body　spirit

not competitive, but suddenly catch fire in the last two miles of a race. There's just something about being surrounded by a mass of humanity, all running or walking pell-mell toward the finish line that impels a person to move faster. I don't know if that means they are competing against the other people or just antagonizing themselves, but finishing a race as fast as you can is a *major* accomplishment. Then when you get past the finishing stage, which is always my overall goal, you bait yourself with improving your race time.

But you don't have to become a runner to experience this thrill. When you think about it, racing is really just a metaphor for life. No matter what fitness activity you choose, no matter what personal goal you set for yourself, you can look at it as if it's a race. And you can get that same thrill of crossing the finish line and the deep sense of personal satisfaction that goes with it when you meet your goals and stick with your program—whether you're walking a treadmill, doing water fitness at the Y, or cycling down a park path.

For me, actual races provide an extra spark—the motivation, the competitive feeling, and the commitment to give my personal best—that helps keep me focused and on track. Plus, races are wonderful social events. Even if you don't want to run, you can still participate. Loads of people walk 5K races, particularly the ones associated with nonprofit causes. These events give you another opportunity to set goals, cross the finish line, and meet lots of supportive people who are out there and committed, just like you are.

I had a race experience recently (August '99) that exemplifies just why I do races. For anyone who has never done a race before, I want to give you the feelings *and* the atmosphere so you will know why it is such a thrill to run or walk and finish.

Pre-race prep

I slept really well the night before and awoke at 5:00am anxious to go! Slipped on my Black Biker/Running Shorts, my Salsa Moving Comfort Bra, my Connectors No More Excuses shirt, Salsa Hat and Salsa Socks. I say, if I can't win any awards, at least I can be fashionable!

After my usual race-day breakfast of a bagel with sugar-free jelly and a banana and a big glass of water, I left my house at 6 am for the drive across the bridge. I zoomed over there in no time and arrived at 7:15 at Connector Debbie's house. Two others were also meeting us. I played my "Rocky" soundtrack CD on the drive over to Debbie's house. As Debbie finished getting her stuff together, I sat on her couch, closed my eyes and visualized my race—seeing myself easily passing each mile mark. Strong. Confident. Seeing the clock with a 59:00.

After the other two people arrived, we piled into my van and headed over to the park, about 4 miles away. We met up with about 10 other Connectors, got our shirts, did the porta-potty thing and walked back to the van to drop off our t-shirts and proceeded to jog back to the starting line to warm up.

The day before, I drank two gallons of water to prepare for the 100-degree temperatures that had maintained all week. When we arrived, it was cool and breezy with a nice cloud cover. I was ONE HAPPY CONNECTOR!

The race

Most of the Connectors started together in the back of the pack. The 5K and the 10K started together. Most of the Connectors were doing the 5K, which was fabulous news for me because there would be all the more Connectors to cheer for me as they waited for me to finish! I always say, the slower you are the more people there are waiting for you, cheering you in.

This race was run almost entirely through beautiful wine vineyards. There was a nice crowd but not overly huge. It took me about 40 seconds to reach the starting line. My goal as with all my 10Ks this year was to finish in under an hour. I had set this goal of running a 10K under an hour way back in July 1997 when I ran my first 5K and watched Debbie run her first 10K under an hour. I was in absolute amazement. How could anyone run so fast? From that day on I would write in detail in my journal about my goal of running a 10K under an hour. Someday...I kept writing, someday. When I ran my first 10K in 1 hour and 27 minutes I knew that big goal would take a while to reach, but since I had seen Debbie, someone I knew, do it, I thought, what the heck, I'll keep chipping away at this big goal. I knew I needed to start out slowly and build from there. So, that's what I did.

Almost immediately I was alone, not in any sort of pack, just alone with my thoughts and visualizations. I flashed back to two years ago when I ran the 5K event. It was at this same race that I had worn shorts in public for one of the very first times (it was extremely hot) and my thighs were rubbing together so much it was killing me (this was before I knew about Body Glide!).

mind body spirit

I had to keep "waking myself up" during this run because it was through the dirt vineyards where the road is very uneven and you can turn your ankle if you're not careful. So I kept looking down and forcing myself to pay attention. I was still basically running alone. There were packs ahead of me and we made a few loops so I knew there were people behind me, but nobody with me. So, I started visualizing various Connectors running by my side. Stride for stride.

By mile 2 the sun popped out and I could feel the ground heating up. During mile 2 to 3 there was a very strong headwind, which was nice on one hand because it was cooling, but because we were on dirt vineyard roads, the pack ahead of me caused a big dust storm in the wind. That was *not fun*. After mile 3 we turned left onto another road so the wind and dust were not a factor anymore. It was at mile 3 that something just clicked for me. I said to myself, "this is the day; I'm going to do it today! Tawni, you're at mile 3, it's time to start picking it up and *go for the gold!* The Connectors are with you. You can do it. Today. Today is the Day!"

So, little by little I started focusing on those runners ahead of me and bringing them closer, little by little. After mile 4, there were a couple of hills and most people were walking up these hills. I seemed to zoom on up them and pass small packs of people. Once over the second hill, I was blessed with a *spectacular* view of the valley. Mile 5 was just down the road after the view. I was hoping to see my friend Debbie at mile 5, but she wasn't there just yet. That's okay, I assured myself, you're doing great and today is the day.

The finish line

One more mile to go. The course turned flat and went back on a paved road and there's an "official lady" who said, ".7 left to go." Just beyond this lady, I saw Connector Debbie and Connector Dani. They started yelling and cheering for me and fell right in line with me. They asked me if I wanted any water, and I just barely managed a shake of my head NO. I was definitely in the "no talk zone." My breathing was very hard and I was huffing and puffing. I knew I had about 1/2 mile to go and I was pretty sure I could run a half-mile in 5 minutes or less, especially with speedster Debbie. I was focusing on the finish line as we made the final turn on the street. Debbie kept saying, "remember 'Velcro Woman'" and "Let's go get this woman, and that one," and "C'mon, you're going way faster than them, we're going to get them up there too."

Debbie knew just what to say. I love the concept of 'Velcro Woman.' It's a mental thing, a way of passing people as you run. You visualize yourself sticking like Velcro to the person in front of you and then pulling away and sticking to the next one. All the time, you're moving forward.

I think I gave her a "snort" here and there, but remained focused on that finish line. I could see the clock turn over to 59 minutes, By now all the CONNECTORS are on the side of the road, YELLING AND JUMPING UP AND DOWN LIKE CRAZY...GO TAWNI. GO GO GO GO TAWNI, GO GO GO GO!

I basically *dove* into the finisher's chute and read my watch: 59:37. The race clock said 1:00:01, which is another good reason to time yourself at races because it takes awhile to get up to the start line.

Wobbly but elated, I leaned on this guy's shoulders as he took me over to the First Aid tent. I assured him "I'm fine; I've just kicked everything out of me and got dizzy when I stopped and my legs kind of buckled out from underneath me." Nope, he took me over to First Aid anyway. The First Aid lady handed me some water, I mumble, "I did it, I did it...I broke an hour. I did it."

After a few minutes, up I went to find the remaining Connectors out on the course, and started running in with them. Life is good! Seeing other Connectors running or walking towards the finish line is the absolute best!

Post race thoughts

I drove an hour and half home, got my logbook out and started reading about this race (5K) from two years ago. Now, the tears flow. The pride I felt from accomplishing this dream goal was overwhelming. I was in awe of myself that I never gave up. Two years of chipping away at this goal, mile by mile, minute by minute, through injuries, no improvements, more injuries, bad races, etc. I never lost sight of this big goal. I thought back to all the times I gave up on myself or never felt worth the effort of even trying because I never followed through on these types of goals in the past.

Through all my ups and downs I would read my logbook and journals and keep thinking about this big goal of "Someday Running a 10K under an hour, Just like Debbie." And so, to have that "same Debbie" run the last half mile of this race with me was simply a dream come true!

mind body spirit

Why do races?

There are many reasons why someone would want to participate in a race. For me and many others, it gives us something to work toward. For me I realized that it is not enough to just decide to run to lose weight. I need-

> "Racing teaches us to challenge ourselves. It teaches us to push beyond where we thought we could go. It helps to find out what we are made of."
>
> PATTISUE PLUMER, U.S. OLYMPIAN

ed to make it more interesting for myself. I also needed to prove to myself that my commitment is real. Races give me that avenue. When I first started racing, it was to just finish. Now, unless I'm doing a marathon, I want to run faster than the last time I ran a race.

Then there is the competitive element. And as I have said, I am definitely competitive. I believe the fastest runners are there for the competition. They want to see how they perform compared to others. I do too!! At the same time, and perhaps more realistically, I want to compete with myself. Besides, anyone who has ever raced can tell you that for some reason they tend to run faster during a race than during a regular training run alone. I think it has to do with the fact that you are competing with everyone else. You want to beat them, even though in reality you probably will not beat most of them.

Each day, before my runs I come to the Connectors for motivation and when the run is done, I share the joy and motivate the next person. I have to say that my best friends are Connectors. We share a common bond. A bond that you can not always find in the people you have in your life. We all want to be fit and will continue to make the connection together. I cherish the gift of the Connectors! Daily I am reminded that there are NO MORE EXCUSES.   BARB, CONNECTING IN NJ

Racing is also a great reason to get together with people of like mind. In other words, it's a great social activity. I know of people who make races a big family event. The whole family comes out—mom, dad, the kids, the grandparents—to offer support to whoever is in the race. It's fun and healthy. For me it's the Connectors I meet, oftentimes for the first time in any given city. We meet, chatter, race together, or at least support each other as cheerleaders on the sidelines. Other people meet new people who happen to enjoy running and share a common interest in racing.

Many times the reason that people walk or run in a race is cause-driven. For instance, one of the best-known races for a cause is called Race for the Cure. Benefiting breast cancer, this is one of the most popular races in the country. Some cities see as many as 50,000 people either running or walking in the event. I have raced in several of these races, including the one in Milwaukee, WI where I ran with Oprah. The interesting thing about this race is that only women can participate. And there is nothing to compare with being in a massive sea of women of all ages, colors, shapes, and sizes, all running together for a good cause.

The Connectors' support was immense, and I found many kindred spirits. Here were women and men, just like me, looking for workout partners, ideas, motivation, support, and validation. I could go on a training run and come back and talk about it with other Connectors who shared all the same ups and downs, fears and questions as me. As I progressed from three miles to five miles to ten miles to a half marathon, the Connectors were there to congratulate me, cheer me on, and share in my every accomplishment. GAYLE, CONNECTING IN CA

The big commitment

When I committed to participate in the Honolulu Marathon in 1997, I didn't know what made me more nervous, training to complete a marathon or trying to raise money for Joints In Motion.

After I sent in my application for the marathon, I was literally sick to my stomach. "What on earth have I done?" I thought. Over and over again I questioned myself. Who the heck did I think I was? I knew for sure I must be crazy and I was setting myself up to fail once again.

But, since ignorance is bliss, I just kept showing up for training and reading everything I could get my hands on about training for a marathon. When I read through Jeff Galloway's advice (www.jeffgalloway.com—Jeff is a world-class marathoner and author of articles and books on long distance running), I thought, "this is doable." Can you imagine? Me, the shape I was in, thinking a marathon was within my grasp? I was always on the sidelines, but now I was experiencing life, participating. The experts kept saying anyone could do a marathon if they'll commit to the training. So that's what I did. Made sure I followed my training schedule. Watched what I ate. Drank a lot of water.

mind body spirit

Looking back on that, one of the first huge goals I committed to, I realize that it was a good thing to be uncertain. Big goals should make us a bit uneasy and nervous! Keeps things interesting! I know I haven't set big enough goals if I'm not a little bit nervous when I commit. Remember: if you shoot for the moon, even if you miss, you'll land among the stars and the view is still very nice!

We met some Maine Connectors for a traditional pasta dinner, and. . . the day of the race, we all met to stretch and at least start together...The sorority feeling of the group was very inspiring. Without recounting the entire race, it was long and emotional for me. Along the way, Connectors were there to cheer me on, unload my extras (Walkman, etc.), and give me toilet paper (which was very meaningful, indeed!). I was not last, but near the back of the pack. My time was poor (in my opinion), 5:27, yet most of the others waited for me at the finish line. Now they either did the relay or the half-marathon, so they must have waited for hours! This was incredible to me.   CAROL, CONNECTING IN MA

Tips for racing

Every race isn't a marathon, but the things that you do to prepare for a five-mile race can be quite similar to what you'd do before a marathon. Here are a few things I have learned that I'll pass on to you in no particular order of importance:

- If you are preparing for a marathon, be sure to fit in at least four to six long runs prior to race day. This means long (four to five hours) runs that simulate the race you are running. The same goes for a shorter race. If you are running a five-mile race for the first time, at least run it a few times before you do the race so that you know what it is like and what your body feels like when you run (or walk, too) that distance.

- Go over the course if possible. For marathons, this can be crucial in planning your "running strategy." It will give you an idea of where the hard spots in the course are (hills) and overall gives your self-confidence a boost to know a little bit more about where you are running. If it's a shorter race, it can be ideal to know the course so that you can plan where to turn on the steam and blaze into the finish line.

- Get used to anything that you will be doing during your race. This means eating and drinking. Don't arrive at race day without having tested what it's like to run and drink water simultaneously. Long races demand that you drink a lot of water and perhaps power up with power gels or an energy bar. Accustom your body to accepting this during your training runs and you will be less likely to be sick during the race, plus you will give your body what it needs to finish strong. Also don't change training habits as far as food and water are concerned when you run the race.

- Rest *means* rest. I know a lot of us (myself included) think, well, I didn't work out today, so that means I have all this energy that I can sweep the garage, rake the yard, vacuum the house, stack the wood, etc. Whoa! Slow down and take it easy, especially in the last week before the race. You'll need all that pent-up energy for your speed burst at the end of the race, as well as just basic endurance during the race.

- Don't break in new shoes on marathon or race day. It's tempting to "start fresh," but if you're going to buy a new pair of shoes, buy a pair about a month before the race and make sure it's a pair that has worked in the past for you or that you have been training in. Surprises for your feet are not what you want when you run your race.

- Drink water about two hours before the race. This starts a cycle where you give your body water and then it starts to demand more as you get into the race. You'll probably end up at the porta-potty right before the race starts, but then you'll be ready to receive water all through the race. I tend to also drink a gallon of extra water in addition to the gallon I already drink daily about 48 hours before a long run or a race over six miles.

- "Carbo-loading" is my favorite part. I eat foods high in carbohydrates that will convert into the glycogen that my body needs during a demanding workout. I do this in the last 48 hours before a race.

"Most people don't plan to fail, but fail to plan," says Harold Shinitzky, a psychologist at Johns Hopkins University School of Medicine. "You should plan long-term goals with short-term steps." Dr. Shinitzky says most people make resolutions without understanding that changing behavior is a process, not a once-a-year activity. "The reality is that change is difficult. You have to figure out how to get there. By implementing certain steps, we can increase the likelihood of achieving our goal."

- Tapering is another thing that people training for long races do. Three weeks before marathon day, run the last long training run and between then and the day of the race do light easy runs. Get extra sleep. Your major runs are behind you and you're resting up so your legs are fresh for the marathon or other race.

- Warm up for the race the same way you warm up for training runs. In other words, keep your little pre-workout ritual the same no matter what. This can act to calm you mentally and you can approach the race as if it were just another run.

- Plan your outfit for the race prior to the day before the race so you are used to it and how it feels. It's fine to buy a new outfit as motivation and a reward for getting to the race, but make sure you have run in it so on race day, you don't discover that the shorts ride up or whatever.

- Eat before you run. I do this anyway, training run or race. I find that if I don't, I can end up with a nauseous feeling during my workout and that can real sap my enthusiasm. Remember, eat early so your body is dealing with digestion at the same time it's dealing with the demands of running.

- Watch your pace. You'll have a trunk load of adrenaline at the beginning of any race, no matter how many times you have run. As a result, you will likely come out too fast, so pull back and slow down. Listen to your body and remember you can always use that extra store of energy later to blaze on by all those other runners who started too fast!

- Focus on the finish. Any pain and fatigue you are going to feel during a race or marathon will likely attack in the later miles. During your long training runs, practice telling yourself, "I can do this distance" or "it's only x number of miles (or minutes)." Your body has a lot more to give than your mind is willing to give it credit for.

Connectors meeting big goals

Here are several inspiring stories I want to share of Connectors who set big goals, achieved them, and changed their lives in the process.

I started by walking 20 minutes a day 4 times a week, adding time and days. I started out by running 30 seconds and walking 5-10 minutes until I was running and jogging and walking and hiking and biking up to an hour a day. My goal was to run a 5K by July 99. Well, on June 20, 1999, I did a 5 mile (8K) in Golden

Gate Park. I was amazed. I started to cry I was so surprised at myself.... I still
don't look like a runner (but I may one day.)   MARY, CONNECTING IN CA

I started a marathon training program in July of 1997. A couple of months into the
program, I decided to enter and run in a local 10K race. Now, I had run in many
5K races (never competitively, always for fun). I had run the distance for the 10K
numerous times, but never in a race situation. The day of the 10K came. I was really
nervous, and was really unsure of whether I could go the distance. Turns out that the
race was mostly for in-line skating, and the 10K race was more of an "afterthought."
There were only about 40 people in the race (including me and my husband).

The gun went off, and off we went. I, of course, was in the back of the pack
running my 11 min +/mile pace. The course was a 2 loop, hilly run on asphalt, and
it was a very warm 75+ southern California day. I rounded my first loop in about
35 minutes. As I came around the bend, I heard the crowd cheering and clapping. To
my chagrin, I realized that most of the runners were FINISHING! I had to stop
and ask a race official where the loop was because I still had one loop to go. After
stopping and going around racers walking across the course who had finished, I was
on my way to my second loop.

About half way through my second loop, I heard footsteps behind me. I was
amazed to see that someone was slower than me! ! There was a middle-aged gentle-
man behind me. I let him catch up to me, and we pushed each other to the finish.
My husband also came back to help me to the finish. Just before reaching the fin-
ish, I asked the man if he would like to enter the chute ahead of me. He gave me a
great big smile and said, "No honey, you go ahead. I am not even in this race. I was
just out running and thought I would check out the course."

When I (FINALLY!) reached the finish line, the crowd was gone, the clock
was stopped and officials were taking down the chute. But I didn't care. I was dead
last, and I didn't care! I was sweaty, thirsty and exhausted, but never in my life
had I felt such exhilaration for being able to finish! I DID IT! I think the man
was an angel, guiding me, giving me hope and faith in myself that I could do it!

CAMILLE, CONNECTING IN CA

Running or walking a race or a complete marathon has given these wonderful and courageous women the thrill of knowing they can do *anything* they
set their minds to. For me the feeling of pride is hard to describe. Reading
about their training runs, week after week. Reading about them getting up

mind body spirit

at 4:30am to get their walks or runs in before the heat got too bad, or braving the elements when its freezing. Listening to them week after week question their sanity for even *dreaming* about doing this. Comforting them when they had bad weeks and felt discouraged and frustrated. Well, I couldn't be more proud if I had run the race or marathon myself. In fact, since I have run a marathon before, and now I've been on the support end, too, I know I had more satisfaction being a cheerleader than in anything I've ever done. Ever. And I've been pretty darn successful in my life (if I do say so myself).

Giving my utmost support to all goal-oriented Connectors taught me the importance of risking, of dreaming big, helping others, and creating an environment where everyone is welcome. All abilities, ages, etc. They all cheer because they all covered the same exact miles. Some faster, some slower, but they all finished. And now this is a new beginning for them, as they realize the doors that open when you don't set limits on what you can do.

On fear of failure

I get asked many times "Aren't you scared the night before a marathon?"

Nope. Nervous and excited but never scared. I trust the training. Isn't it funny how calm you can be when you know you've done everything to bring you to where you are? Nervous energy is great. I just think of it as "speedy energy vibes." Then they say, "But aren't you scared you won't finish?" Nope. I've done the training. And if for some reason I wasn't able to finish that would be upsetting to me, but it's the *journey* and all I've learned to get me to that starting line. It sure helps that I've done a lot of races and have always finished. But if ever I can't, I'll cross that bridge when it happens, certainly no need to be scared about "What If."

About two years ago I was 150 pounds overweight, the mother of three, and miserable. I found myself moving numbly through each day, just trying to get by. Finally I thought, it's my life: mine to shape, to throw away, to seize hold of, to waste, or to celebrate. I began to walk and the simple act of demanding the time to do this changed my whole perspective. I began to take a look at my eating habits, which were self-destructive. I began to lose weight: 100 pounds in one year. Now I walk four miles a day and have goals like hiking nine miles on local nature trails with friends. I'll never be that frozen, overweight lump of a woman again. After all, it's my life!   CATHEY, CONNECTING IN WI

In my past fear paralyzed me and so I basically never did anything because I was a worrier and just too afraid to try anything. Well, that was the big waste of time. The other biggest waste of time was "waiting till I got thin" to participate in life! I'll never get those years back. I can live and participate now, but all those opportunities that kept coming my way and I just kept saying no. I had tons and tons of excuses, but basically I was just too afraid of trying and failing.

Commitment to train for life

I think it was Henry Ford who once said something to the effect that "There are those who say they can, and there are those who say they can't, and they're both right." My greatest hope is that you will be one of those people who will say "I can!" There are four principles I want you to take to heart and apply to your life as you train for life:

1 **Make a commitment.**

   You must decide in your heart and in your mind that your life is changed forever, from this point forward. You are no longer the person you have been. You are committed to looking at life differently and living your life differently.

   You will not allow any excuses to interfere with your new heartfelt and mental decision to be a different person. You won't say, "Well, I'll make changes in my life after the new year," or "Once I've paid off my bills" or "After my divorce is final." or "After I've moved." or a zillion other excuses. Because the moment an excuse popped into your head, you are not ready to change your life. It's just that simple. Accordingly, your life will more than likely continue as it always has.

2 **Make it real.**

   Once you have made a commitment, this next step is not impossible. Making your commitment real means to take steps to make some real, tangible changes in your life. This is where you apply the ten steps of training for life. By observing even some of these steps you are doing something; you are making your commitment real. For example, when I first started to make a change in my life, the two most challenging parts of the process were getting up early to work out, and trying to drink up to eight glasses of water each day. In some ways, the water was harder to do than the workouts. So, I started small, with baby steps. I started by drinking up to three glasses of water each day for the first week and then four glasses each day for

mind body spirit

another week, and so on until I reached the optimal level. But the fact that I did *something* made my commitment real.

The trouble is that if you don't make a true heart and mind commitment, you cannot make it real. You will simply not be able to stick with it. You will have to go back to principle #1 above.

3 Set goals and achieve them.

You must set goals for yourself. This should become an almost routine part of your life. The ten steps to train for life are all a number of goals. These are goals you should try to incorporate into your daily life. Working out, drinking enough water, making smart food choices, recommitting yourself daily, are all goals that add up to one big achievement over time. But you should also make other goals. For my fitness program I include upcoming races as goals to train for.

My goals are to not only complete the race, but to outperform myself. In the process I instill in myself discipline, confidence, a sense of purpose, focus, etc. This, in turn, has resulted in performing more effectively in other areas of my life. I'm not as afraid as I used to be about trying new things, of having new experiences, of meeting new people, and so on. I am now setting goals and achieving things I never before thought possible.

4 Give yourself credit.

When I achieve a goal, particularly a goal that I had previously considered impossible for me to achieve, I have learned to celebrate my achievement. I give myself credit. True, I may not have arrived at that accomplishment as quickly, or as efficiently, or impressively as someone else might. But I give myself credit for what I have done. I try not to compare myself to others. Obviously, I can't run a marathon in two-and-half-hours, but I know I can run a marathon. It is something I did. And because I did it, I know it is something I can do and I am proud of my achievement.

The lesson here is that you can get yourself to do something. You have adopted the right frame of mind, you have made an effort to work towards a goal, and you have reached your goal. Training for life is incorporating all this into your daily life. You don't just do it on nice days (like my fair weather running friends) or at times when you just feel like it. You make an ongoing concerted, consistent effort, all the time, even when you don't really feel like it.

CHAPTER 8

Food 101

> *I can't figure out why I'm struggling to stay alive. It takes effort, so much effort and I'm just too tired to care. I bought bags of candy to hand out to my customers and have already gone through one whole bag of Butterfingers. Why did I ever buy the candy to begin with? Who am I kidding? I can't believe I've let myself get so FAT. It seems all-consuming and I know I've given up and I just can't seem to find my way back. I swore I'd never get above 200 pounds and now 300 is becoming a reality. I pray I'll have the strength and discipline to stop this cycle of bingeing and depression.*

> JOURNAL ENTRY, OCTOBER 28, 1995

For me, food became less about what I ate and more about how much I ate. But for some people that isn't true. You can look at food in terms of your lifestyle changes in two ways. I call these two ways the tortoise and the hare. Most people go for the hare method of doing things. One example of this is the desire to win a lottery and instantly be rich, without any of the effort or hard work that goes into achieving wealth. Now perhaps that's everyone's fantasy (and I admit I have let myself go there a few times in my life), but look at the odds. And you aren't even in control of whether you win the lottery or not; it's all up to chance. But you still buy your lottery ticket and hope for some instant gratification.

I parallel the lottery idea with someone who just wants to take one of the many pills that are now being touted today to lose weight. I have to laugh when I hear commercials saying if you just take this pill you can avoid all that "sweaty exercise." I was there once myself, hoping that some pill or some diet would be the answer to my problems with weight. What I didn't realize was that it was about much more than just food.

Now for the tortoise, which I basically became three-plus years ago. As you read in the fable, he plods slowly along while his opponent takes the fast, apparently easy path to victory. He has many obstacles but nevertheless always pushes forward and eventually wins the race. Like anything else worth doing or having, it took work for him to finally cross the finish line.

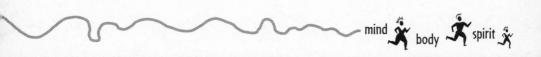

mind   body   spirit

To me, the tortoise represents the exercise and changes in your food choices that you make along your path to fitness and health. You see small successes along the way, perhaps nothing like the fireworks of a lottery winner, but success is success! In this case, life is not a race; it's a journey and it's the journey that is important.

Eating right

When you're trying to eat right, picture yourself with a halo of words around your head. The words read, "lower in fat and sugar, high in fiber, variety." If you wear this food halo, you truly will be eating like a good food "angel." Eating this way means a balance of the four food groups you learned about in first grade. In case first grade was a while ago for you, there are now five food groups instead of four: meats, dairy products, fruits, vegetables, and breads and cereals.

Here are some of the things I say to myself about eating healthy:
• If I'm tempted to eat something that isn't good for me: Have you eaten your three servings of vegetables and two servings of fruit yet? If not, you can't have that (usually a carbo product) until you do.
• When I'm not that hungry, but see something that is tempting to eat: You're not on a diet. You don't have to have X today. You can have it tomorrow when you really are hungry. It will still be there.
• If you eat that, it will interfere with the way you feel when you work out.
• If I'm eating too quickly: Stop eating for a couple of minutes and see if your body really needs anything more to eat.   ELIZABETH, CONNECTING IN CA

I have often been asked, Tawni, do you ever "cheat" on your diet? The answer is, I'm not on a diet, so I don't ever cheat. Diets are about a phase. They're about trying to get a fast fix on a problem that defies fast fixes. I do my best each day to eat what is good for me and I am constantly trying to better myself in terms of my nutrition—and I still have a ways to go! No, I don't eat whatever I want, because that's how I got to be 275 pounds. I will say that what I want has changed since I have made a commitment to my new lifestyle. Food has lost most of its romance for me. It's now about being hungry and nourishing my soul. This didn't happen for me overnight. And I still have my days. It's not important what point you're at; we all start somewhere and we all struggle with certain things.

Another facet of eating right is reading labels at the grocery store. Why bother? You are striving to eat a diet rich in whole grains, vegetables and fruit along with lean dairy and protein. Some fat should be added and sweets, or anything else for that matter, shouldn't be forbidden, but rather balanced in your diet.

One Connector writes to me:

My problem is a balanced diet. At one point in my life (read 20s), I was borderline anorexic and now at the age of 49 I still experience the thoughts, etc. that go along with this disease. I still have problems with social eating and eating in general. For the past 2 weeks I have been living on rice cakes, ju jubes, cereal, etc. Don't know what this is all about. Any hints about getting around this would be greatly appreciated. Every morning I tell myself that this is the day I will eat properly but what I am doing right now? Sucking on a butterscotch candy. I am not overweight but was chubby as a kid and of course was kidded about that all those many years ago. It just never leaves you, Tawni. Now I weigh about 105 lbs. but have the old image of "fat." I have been for counseling for this and am a lot better but every once in awhile it will lift its ugly head. That is where I have been for the last month. When I do eat, it's at the worst possible time — 10-11:00 at night for goodness sake.

DIANNE, CONNECTING IN CANADA

My advice to Dianne is the same that I would give to anyone coming to me with this challenge. Continue counseling with a health professional and start with one baby step. Your one baby step in this case might be to eat one vegetable a week. Just one carrot for the first week. The next week, try another vegetable, say, one floret of broccoli dipped in some fat free ranch dressing. We create our own habits and that means we can also change them. Introduce your body to something healthy so it will start calling for that instead of the empty calories you have been feeding it.

Another thing about this kind of situation is to ask yourself that very important question: am I really hungry or is there something else going on in my life? Am I tired, sad, angry, insecure, frustrated, or what? That can usually help you solve that eating late at night problem. And when you are hungry late at night, eat a piece of fruit. The calories are low and the fill factor is high.

mind body spirit

Americans are slowly changing their eating patterns toward healthier diets. However, a considerable gap remains between recommended dietary patterns and what Americans actually eat.

· Only 27% of women and 19% of men eat the recommended five or more servings of fruits and vegetables each day.

Although the amounts of total fat, saturated fatty acids, and cholesterol that Americans consume have decreased, they remain above recommended levels for a large proportion of the population.

· Between 20% and 30% of the nation's adults are at least 30 pounds overweight, and more than 3 million women weigh at least 100 pounds more than their recommended body weight.

Like adults, many young people in the United States make poor eating choices.

· More than 84% of young people eat too much fat, and less than 30% eat the recommended number of servings of fruits and vegetables each day.

· Nearly 25% of young people aged 6-17 years are considered overweight. The percentage of young people who are seriously overweight has more than doubled in the last 30 years.

CENTERS FOR DISEASE CONTROL, NATIONAL CENTER FOR CHRONIC DISEASE PREVENTION AND HEALTH PROMOTION, NUTRITION AND PHYSICAL ACTIVITY REPORT, 11/99

Appetite

As you work out regularly, you will notice that your appetite will change. Aerobic exercise affects something in your body called the "appestat." This is your body's natural automatic appetite control, but if you are inactive or have the tendency to eat a lot of food all the time, your appestat is thrown off. It basically gets broken and doesn't know when you should eat and when you shouldn't. The miraculous thing about exercise is that it will actually get your appestat back on track. You will find that your eating habits start to adjust based on your exercise. Your body will demand certain things that you burn off during your workout—vitamins, minerals, protein, carbohydrates, etc.

Fat & calories

Remember, trying to lose fat by not eating as much but running or walking more won't work. Keep in mind the way your metabolism works. Not giving your body the fuel that it needs and demanding that it give you the performance that you want when you work out will make your body grab on to the fat stores that it has and hold on for dear life! It's like anything else; keep your exercising and eating habits in balance.

I suggest that you exercise in the morning, have three balanced meals and supplement yourself with healthy snacks throughout the day. Don't let your body get to the point that we all do when we are busy—that we are so hungry we feel sick! Keep giving your body small quantities of food during the day and you won't be as tempted to overeat at a particular meal, like dinner.

Obviously you have read and heard enough about calories that you know the simple fact that eating more calories than you get rid of will prevent you from losing weight. And you haven't come this far just to sit around!

The other key thing about calories is that because you have started to be more aware of what you are putting in your mouth, you will begin to train yourself to think "are these calories that I actually *want?*" It goes beyond "calories" and gets to the real issue, which is why I want it.

Effective eating for athletes

Athletes need to eat effectively to perform well, but it applies to everyone who wants to make a lifestyle change. Both athletes and sedentary people would benefit from eating more fruits, vegetables, and whole grains (complex carbs) and moderate amounts of lean dairy, protein and some fat. I personally take a vitamin supplement (One A Day plus Iron—check with your doctor before taking any supplement to get the one that's right for you) to round out my vitamin and mineral needs, but I strive to get most of what I need from raw, basic foods.

When and what to eat

An ideal food fuel-up for me right before a run or race is something small. I eat a bagel with jelly and a banana and drink a big glass of water. If you're out the door in the morning, a small glass of orange juice or a few bites of an energy bar may settle your morning hunger pangs, but only if your body can handle that. For me, anything that I eat the day of the race or run is simple and bland. For you it might be something different. Do you feel you have a better workout with no food beforehand? A sizeable breakfast two hours before? Experiment and find out what your body needs in terms of performance.

What about sports bars, gels & drinks?

Although a billion-dollar business is done each year in sports fluids, energy bars, and other sports "supplements," in most cases, what your body needs most is an ample amount of nutritious foods, nothing in excess. The food you eat doesn't *have* to be specially created for athletes, as long as you are providing your body with adequate fuel in relation to the exercise demands you are placing on it.

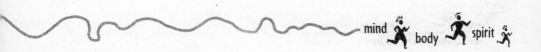

mind body spirit

Before Exercise/Competition

Two to 6 hours before an endurance event, depending on individual preference, a meal providing 85 to 200 g carbohydrates should be consumed. Food choices should provide mainly complex carbohydrates and should be low in fat and protein. Athletes should choose foods that are familiar and comforting, have been consumed before training sessions, and are known not to cause gastric distress. Athletes should not experiment with new foods or beverages on competition day. A liquid meal supplement that provides a balance of fluid and nutrients may be helpful for athletes with pre-competition jitters and gastric distress.

Five to 10 minutes before exercise or competition, fluids containing a small amount of carbohydrate may be consumed to maintain blood glucose level. There does not appear to be a significant insulin rebound effect from this practice, although some athletes do not tolerate this comfortably.

During Exercise/Competition

Small carbohydrate feedings during endurance events of more than 1 hour may delay fatigue. Feedings should be at regular intervals to provide about 24g carbohydrates every 30 minutes. Athletes should become comfortable with these feedings during their practice sessions. Athletes often find that consumption of carbohydrate-containing sport beverages is better tolerated than solid foods during activity. Athletes should consume fluid on a fixed time schedule during activity, regardless of thirst.

After Exercise/Competition

Carbohydrate consumption after exercise ensures repletion of muscle glycogen. Research shows that muscle will replete glycogen stores to a higher degree when up to 600 g easily digestible carbohydrate is consumed within the first several hours after exercise. The athlete should begin eating high-carbohydrate foods as soon as possible after physical exertion. Blood glucose, insulin, and glycogen synthetase levels will remain elevated to promote glycogen synthesis and replete the muscle reserves

PAPER ON THE POSITION OF THE AMERICAN DIETETIC ASSOCIATION AND THE CANADIAN DIETETIC ASSOCIATION: NUTRITION FOR PHYSICAL FITNESS AND ATHLETIC PERFORMANCE FOR ADULTS, 1999 PERMISS@EATRIGHT.ORG

This is not to say that a so-called "energy" bar cannot be a convenient mid-morning snack, especially if you have worked out pretty hard earlier in the morning. Energy bars can supply fuel for our bodies, but I wouldn't advise *living* on energy bars. For one thing, it would get too boring and for another, you'll be depriving your body of the variety it naturally yearns for in food.

If you are racing on a particularly hot or humid day, you may choose to tank up on a sports drink such as Gatorade. Of course your water intake is also important, but that should be a daily thing anyway.

As far as gels go, I do use them during marathons and I find that they really do seem to work, giving your muscles an added "power infusion." They're not my favorite things in the world to eat, but I just sort of suck them down and follow that with a lot of water.

Post-exercise fuel-up

The great part about finishing a race is that we get to eat afterwards and not feel the slightest bit guilty! After a long, exhausting race, you need a diet high in carbohydrates to replace what your muscles have lost during the exertion. Good snacks include but are not limited to a dry bagel with jelly, pasta, a banana, carrots, and yogurt. Energy bars are also good if they are low in fat. Of course, if I have just run a marathon, I have eaten energy bars throughout the race and am usually sick to death of those things by the time I finish!

Food & stress

Ah, stress. You say that to 10 different people and it will mean 10 different things, plus each person will have a different way of dealing with the chaos. The question is how do you avoid eating everything in sight when you seem to have the perfect reason to? For me, logging what I eat really makes me aware of what I put in my mouth every day. It makes me think and it keeps me balanced. I also keep "junk" out of my house, like ice cream or whatever else is tempting me with its high-fat content. Instead, I keep carrots and other veggies cut up and stored in the fridge for quick munching.

If the stress gets really bad, I go to my favorite restaurant and eat what I am yearning for (within reason), but I confine it to one meal. I don't let it take over my life. This is about changing the way you live for the rest of your life, not just getting through today and not worrying about tomorrow.

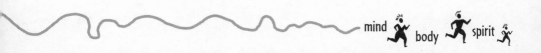

mind body spirit

I guarantee that there will be some sort of stress in your life pretty much the whole way through. I can also guarantee that even after you eat whatever it is you try to tell yourself you need at the time, the stress will still be there, now accompanied by the hallowed voice of guilt.

So I stop myself and say, what is it that you really want? Do you want attention, reassurance, power? Do you really just need a hug or an encouraging word? Training your mind to ask your body these types of questions can help take away the craving.

Habits

In the last three years, I have had to battle my ingrained habits enough times that I finally reached for the dictionary. After all, what was it that I was really fighting? Habits are patterns of behavior based on repetition. That was a "light bulb" moment for me. As I stood there in my apartment with a worn copy of Webster's Dictionary held loosely in one hand, I realized that the beauty of habits is that *we defined them. We* make the *choices* that *become* habits. Knowing that is so powerful.

When I first started making the connection, the best I could do was to order a medium pizza instead of a large one, or a pint of ice cream instead of a quart. That's the best that I could do at the time. Those were the baby steps that I could make. Now, if I'm out and I feel like going to Dairy Queen, I have a small serving of their non-fat yogurt. This is not about going without; it's about making compromises and that is life.

I'd just had to buy size 42 men's jeans because my size 22 women's jeans were too tight in the legs and the stores didn't seem to have any size 24s. I started Weight Watchers and got out my old copy of Make the Connection. *This time I was determined to do it. But I wasn't going to tell anybody just yet. I didn't like being noticed when I was just beginning to try to succeed. If people knew that I was trying some would take it upon themselves to monitor, question, advise, and request justification for my choices. I didn't need that added stress. I needed, first and foremost, to get my eating under control, get a handle on sweet bingeing, and to begin making better food choices a habit. I would exercise when I felt like it but not torture myself. I would concentrate on nutrition first—I had far fewer excuses to overcome for my eating habits than for my exercise habits.* FLORENCE, CONNECTING IN CA

Food & the holidays

For most of us, the holidays are the most challenging times of the year. This is when so many people fall off track in the face of all that temptation. I have some tips that may help you stay focused on your health and fitness goals.

- Don't buy Halloween candy (or Easter candy or Christmas candy). Period. If I'm going to be home for Halloween, I buy sugarless bubble gum to hand out. Don't fool yourself and buy candy "for the kids." Or buy something you hate. I can't stand coconut, so if I was "forced" to buy candy, I would buy something that had coconut in it. One year I even gave out toothbrushes. I don't play the game; I know I won't have the willpower to not eat it, so I just don't buy it instead of trying to fool myself.

- I try and get all my Christmas shopping done early. What does this have to do with food? Plenty! There are so many activities going on during the Thanksgiving and Christmas holidays that if you aren't stressing out about buying last-minute gifts, you'll be less likely to feed your face too much.

- I give lots of gift certificates. They're easy and fast, and give everyone the chance to get just what he or she wants. Magazine subscriptions are an especially good gift idea because they are fast and keep giving each month of the year.

- Remember there are ways to cook large meals like Thanksgiving and Christmas dinner and substitute low- or non-fat items in your main dishes. For instance, you can make mashed potatoes with 99% fat-free chicken broth instead of using butter. In addition, I suggest that you plan for your success. Bring something that means that you are taking care of yourself instead of using the meal as an excuse to overeat.

I don't cook, but I do make great reservations! My mom never cooked and I guess I missed that lesson along the way. What I will do is bring a salad and a veggie platter with me wherever I go. That way I know there will at least be something healthy for me to eat. Also, I bring my workout clothes and shoes and I *always* take a walk before and after the meal, usually with some member of the family. We spend that time sharing a good walk and conversation *away* from all the food. I tell the family/friends ahead of time to bring something to walk in and we'll go for a walk before and after the meal. It's always my favorite part of the day.

mind 🏃 body 🏃 spirit 🏃

"I deserve NOT to eat that" helped me a lot, and it's helping now. We tend to feel deprived when eating right and want to treat ourselves with a piece of cake or a few cookies. It's not a treat if it is hurting our bodies and our confidence. When I am tempted, I say out loud, "I deserve not to have that," and get the temptation out of sight. It really does help, because I have turned giving up one thing into giving myself something better. It turns a negative into a positive. CHRYSTAL, CONNECTING IN MN

The other thing I've done, for instance at Thanksgiving, is go around the table and share what I'm most grateful for. And I usually volunteer at a church or shelter by serving meals to those less fortunate and it reminds me of all that I have. I bring all the leftovers from my dinner to the shelter so I won't have to battle the urge to continue my holiday meal long after the holiday is over.

Start now by creating a new tradition. Some years I've gone out to eat and that's been great too. Our family was never too big on huge traditions. So, I've done different things different years. For Thanksgiving I honestly think of it as a Thursday dinner. I don't put all the pressure of "Thanksgiving" on myself. I eat 3 meals that day and 2 snacks just as I do every other day of the year.

I focus on seeing friends and family and not on how much food I can eat that day. Don't get me wrong, before I started making the connection, I was stuffed more than the Thanksgiving turkey, always miserable afterwards wishing I wouldn't have. So, there's really nothing that will be on the table this year that I haven't had a million times before. So, why bother? I eat like a person who respects herself and her body.

Alcohol

Some of you may remember from your college days that after a heavy-duty party the night before, you wake up feeling sluggish, drowsy, like you didn't get enough rest. You can barely force your limbs to move their usual way. Guess what? It hasn't changed. And worse, when you are a walker or runner who demands extra from your body, alcohol can affect your performance.

I'm not going to advocate total abstinence because I don't like the pressure of having to be "perfect," but I do advise that you take into consideration the effects of alcohol not only on your workout, but also on your body in general. Everyone likes to have a glass of bubbly on New Year's or a glass of beer once a month or twice a year. The key is not overdoing it because not only are you absorbing extra calories from the alcohol; you're also slowing yourself down for no good reason.

The nighttime munchies

I usually eat dinner at six, so around nine or nine-thirty in the evening, I can get the munchies. I don't like the way it feels to be hungry or to be deprived, but sometimes I will tell myself, just go to bed. Now this can work. I can fall asleep and be able to eat the next morning before I go for my run. But perfection's halo doesn't hang over my head! One thing I do to combat this is have a glass of water. The down side is that I end up peeing in the middle of the night. So most of the time I eat a piece of fruit like an apple or a few teaspoons of yogurt. It's simply the act of putting something in your stomach to stave off that growling and gurgling that's keeping the neighborhood awake.

My father was a preacher. My mother, who had six children in seven years, was a housewife. It was really the only choice she had with so many little ones around. My mom always tried to do what was right. Doing what was right, at that time, included cleaning your plate. Despite the fact that I was a young child, I learned this lesson early. During my senior year of high school and my first two years of college, I became bulimic. After I got married and had a wonderful husband and family, I wanted to lose weight and tried just about every diet there was. I would always end up rationalizing by saying that I was happy the way I was. But even that came to a grinding halt. I finally got tired of saying, I'll try tomorrow when I knew that my mind and body wouldn't.

When I found the Connectors, I rejoiced to know that whenever I went for a walk, it mattered to someone out there. Once again I am losing my pound or two a week consistently, without the help of diets or pills. It's just a matter of eating right and exercising.   CANDY, CONNECTING IN CO

My way of eating

I could spend pages telling you about meal days. But what I really want you to know is that I do my best every day to follow the food group guidelines. I think everyone's nutrition undergoes fine-tuning daily; I know mine does because it's sure not perfect! I like to keep the ol' food pyramid in mind.

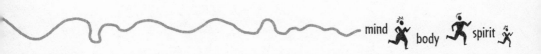

mind 🏃 body 🏃 spirit 🏃

Remember the food guide pyramid? You see it everywhere these days. The pyramid is just a graph that shows the relative proportions of what types of foods you should include in your daily meals. Complex carbohydrates — grains, veggies, and fruits — form both the pyramid's foundation and the foundation of your new eating plan.

Food Guide Pyramid

A Guide to Daily Food Choices

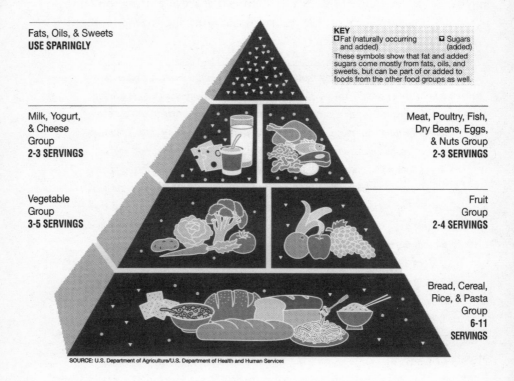

Fats, Oils, & Sweets
USE SPARINGLY

KEY
☐ Fat (naturally occurring and added)   ◪ Sugars (added)
These symbols show that fat and added sugars come mostly from fats, oils, and sweets, but can be part of or added to foods from the other food groups as well.

Milk, Yogurt,
& Cheese
Group
2-3 SERVINGS

Meat, Poultry, Fish,
Dry Beans, Eggs,
& Nuts Group
2-3 SERVINGS

Vegetable
Group
3-5 SERVINGS

Fruit
Group
2-4 SERVINGS

Bread, Cereal,
Rice, & Pasta
Group
**6-11
SERVINGS**

SOURCE: U.S. Department of Agriculture/U.S. Department of Health and Human Services

Use the Food Guide Pyramid to help you eat better every day. . .the Dietary Guidelines way. Start with plenty of Breads, Cereals, Rice, and Pasta; Vegetables; and Fruits. Add two to three servings from the Milk group and two to three servings from the Meat group.

Each of these food groups provides some, but not all, of the nutrients you need. No one food group is more important than another — for good health you need them all. Go easy on fats, oils, and sweets, the foods in the small tip of the Pyramid.

Don't be fooled by low-fat foods

According to an October 13, 1999 report in the *Journal of the American Medical Association,* the majority of adult Americans who are trying to lose weight aren't cutting calories *and* exercising simultaneously. Don't be pulled into the low-fat food trap! Losing weight is not about just avoiding fattening foods because low-fat foods can more than make up for the calories in high fat foods since we tend to eat *more* of the low-fat foods, figuring they're not as bad for us. Instead adjust your food portions so that you are eating smaller amounts of food; this in turn will lead to better food choices overall since you will force yourself to think about how much and what is going into your mouth.

In the kitchen

I can personally attest to not wanting to spend a lot of time in the kitchen since I spend almost *no* time in the kitchen! But for those of you looking to reduce the time you do spend cooking healthy, I offer this advice. Use a shopping list (to keep you on track and away from all those tempting high-calorie, less healthy foods) and keep a well-stocked kitchen. The National Institute of Health and its affiliates encourages you to "read the labels as you shop and pay attention to serving size and servings per container. Compare the total calories in similar products and choose the lowest calorie ones." Good advice!

Reading labels for health

One of the big goals you're going to want to set for yourself is to begin eating a well-balanced diet that includes whole grains, fruits and vegetables. You don't have to become a scientist or even a dietician to learn how to choose healthy foods, but you do have to learn how to read the labels.

The FDA has strict guidelines for the types of labels manufacturers can use to describe their products (low, lite, free) and the heath claims they can make (such as "may reduce the risk of heart disease or osteoporosis"). For a great crash course in how to read labels and understand those nutrition facts on cans and boxes, check out the American Heart Association web site (www.deliciousdecisions.org/sm/fle.html) for a good, solid discussion of what those labels and the percentages actually mean. This clever online notebook also includes loads of shopping and cooking tips for making the switch to low-fat, healthy eating.

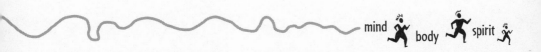

mind body spirit

But just to give you a head start, here are some basics. Assume that you're looking at containers of sour cream and you're wondering about the fat content. The carton labeled "Free" contains the least amount. Cartons labeled "Very Low" and "Low" have a little bit more. Cartons labeled "Reduced" or "Less Fat" contain even more—but at least 25% of the fat has been removed.

Healthful guidelines

Five major health organizations have endorsed the Unified Dietary Guidelines. The American Cancer Society, the American Dietetic Association, the American Academy of Pediatrics, the American Heart Association, the American Society for Clinical Nutrition and the National Institutes of Health all agree now on a single plan for healthy eating:

- Eat a variety of foods.
- Choose most of what you eat from plant sources. More than half— 55 percent or more—of your daily calories should come from carbohydrates like grains, fruits, and vegetables. Eat five or more servings of fruits and vegetables and six or more servings of bread, pasta, rice and cereal every day.
- Limit high-fat foods, especially those from animal sources. No more than 10 percent of your calories should come from saturated fat and no more than 30 percent of your total calories should from all types of fat.
- Limit cholesterol to 300 milligrams or less each day (less than the amount in two eggs).
- Cut down your salt intake to 6 grams (about one teaspoon) or less per day.
- Eat simple sugars in moderation.

There are different types of fat-saturated, polyunsaturated, and mono-unsaturated. Your body needs a certain amount of dietary fat to work efficiently, but the average person eats way more fat than the minimal amount your body needs. The most trouble comes from saturated fat, the kind in foods from animal sources, such as meat, whole dairy products, and the so-called "tropical oils" (coconut oil, palm oil, and palm kernel oil).

Since food labels identify fat content and the type of fat (along with other important things like cholesterol and sodium), you can use these labels to help you plan your menus to follow the Unified Dietary Guidelines.

Food to keep in your house

Shopping for quick, low-fat food items? Fill your kitchen cupboards with low calorie basics like the following:

- Fat free or low fat milk, yogurt, cheese, and cottage cheese
- Light or diet margarine
- Eggs/egg substitutes
- Sandwich breads, bagels, pita bread, English muffins
- Soft corn tortillas, low fat flour tortillas
- Low fat, low sodium crackers
- Plain cereal, dry or cooked
- Rice, pasta
- White meat chicken or turkey (remove skin)
- Fish and shellfish (not battered)
- Beef: round, sirloin, chuck arm, loin and extra lean ground beef
- Pork: leg, shoulder, tenderloin
- Dry beans and peas
- Fresh, frozen, canned fruits in light syrup or juice
- Fresh, frozen, or no salt added canned vegetables
- Low fat or nonfat salad dressings
- Mustard and catsup
- Jam, jelly, or honey
- Herbs and spices
- Salsa

(Source for above: The National Heart, Lung, and Blood Institute in cooperation with the National Institute of Diabetes and Digestive and Kidney Diseases, National Institutes of Health.)

Restaurant eating

I find that one of the most common things people tell me is that they can't eat out when they're "dieting" or trying to lose weight. I find that so hard to believe! I mean, we're not talking about sacrificing for a little while; this is your life! You're not going to "never go out to a restaurant again." So why do it now? Instead, let's think about changing the way we eat when we are at a restaurant. It is a mindset and believe me, you can learn it.

mind body spirit

You can start by choosing the places that you go to eat. A seafood place is probably going to be easier to make leaner choices at than a Mexican food restaurant, but there are possibilities there, too. When you are first starting out, you may want to check a restaurant out first before you end up there. You may choose to avoid some restaurants because it's harder to set yourself up for success in them.

Qualifying a Healthy Choice in Restaurants & Food

Will your restaurant choice pass the healthy eater's test?

· Serves butter alternatives like margarine or bean dip

· Can substitute skim milk for whole, two percent or cream

· Serves lean slices of meat and chicken (trimmed of fat)

· Can have heavy sauces, dressings, or gravy on the side

· Emphasizes the happiness of its patrons by filling special requests

· Offers a specific "light" or "heart healthy" menu

Once it passes my test, I seek out foods that fall into one of these healthy categories.

· Steamed

· Fresh (as in, from the garden)

· Broiled

· Poached

· Roasted

· Baked

· Lightly sautéed or stir-fried (with a minimum of oil)

No matter where I am, I first read the menu back and front. I read all the ingredients in their dishes and I mentally start figuring out what ingredients they have in the kitchen. If there's a dish with marinara sauce, but I want to have something that is originally prepared in a cream sauce, I know that they can swap sauces for me.

If I am interested in something other than a pasta dish, then I think, now how would they prepare that? If I can't figure it out myself, I ask. Not surprisingly, I am often told, "oh, that's sautéed in butter" or "that's marinated overnight in olive oil." I have gotten into a habit of creating my own menu. If a pasta dish that sounds interesting to me is good in every way and then is covered in cream sauce, I ask the waitress if there is another way we can prepare that. If it's a chicken breast, then is it served with the skin on or off? Of course, you prefer it *off*. Always feel free to find out how a dish is prepared and served.

Let's say that the office is going out for Mexican food (assume your vote to get sandwiches was outvoted). There's a great trick you can do in Mexican restaurants to head off one of the worst things about just sitting down at the table: ask the waitress not to bring chips to the table. If you're with a group of people, ask them to keep the chips on their side of the table, away from you. In terms of the rest of the menu, I order black beans instead of refried (or find out how the refried beans are prepared). I hold the sour cream and the guacamole. I order rice, which is filling, and spicy chicken. Salsa is fat-free in most cases. Soft corn tortillas are also a good lower fat alternative.

See? It's just a matter of learning what is healthy and what is not. People sometimes tell me that they don't know how to order when they go out. This just blows me away! There are enough books on what foods are fattening and which ones aren't out there to fill several warehouses! The best advice I can give you is to learn what foods are healthy and then *ask for what you want.*

Dealing with the fast food habit

Another aspect of our society of instant gratification has to do with our rushing from place to place or only having 30 minutes for lunch, etc. Approached the right way, you will see that there is no excuse for not eating healthy, even in the face of these fast food chains with their enticing smells of greasy fries and sizzling hamburgers. I know from experience that you can get into the habit of making work such a priority that eating becomes just another chore rather than something we do for our bodies.

My advice for breaking your fast food habit is to start with one small step at a time. First look at how much fast food you eat per week. Do you take four trips to your nearest burger joint during the week? Order three pizzas from the nearby pizza place? Work on cutting back, slowly and realistically. Tell yourself—and write this in your journal or on your wish list if it helps—this week I will only go to "x" burger place three times instead of four. And change your selections. Order a side salad with low fat dressing. Try the broiled or grilled chicken breast sandwich with barbecue sauce instead of the big cheeseburger. Order your pizza with vegetables, not extra cheese. These are baby food steps. Meanwhile you will be doing a baby exercise step as well; maybe you'll be walking around the block for ten minutes one day a week.

October 1998, 188 pounds
Learned to take snacks with me in the car—apples, raisins, and grapes. That kept me from feeling deprived and kept me from responding to external food cues like passing Burger King and other restaurants when traffic was slow and smells from the bakery at work—I work at the county jail and the bakery is right next to the employee entrance. If I had my afternoon snack right after work, then I was not tempted to stop for unplanned food.   FLORENCE, CONNECTING IN TX

---

mind body spirit

On the road in fast food America

If you're like most of us, when you pack the car and hit the road, you expect that the food fare along the way isn't going to be too healthy. But you just accept that as part of the road trip. Nothing you can do about it, right?

Wrong! I'll admit that convenience or fast food is one of the greatest challenges for anyone trying to achieve fitness, health, and nutrition goals. Pulling off the interstate to the nearest fast food establishment is fast and easy.

The key to getting around the lure of fast food is proper planning. While it may be easier to pull in to the nearest fast food restaurant, the healthful food choices can be very limited. So I avoid these detours from my fitness and health goals. Here's an example of how I manage to combine travel and sound nutrition.

Tawni's terrific trip

What follows are my journal notes from my trip driving down to Southern California for the 1999 Thanksgiving holiday weekend. When I weighed in Monday morning after the four-day weekend, I weighed less than when I left to start the holiday weekend. I can attest that success feels better than fast food tastes any day! And, as you'll see, a lot of it's in the planning.

> *Tuesday, November 23 (the night before I was to leave):*
> *Grocery shopping: baby carrots (prepackaged in a small bag), apples, bananas, energy bars, non-fat ranch salad dressing. I packed my suitcase and had everything ready to go for Wednesday morning. Packed my cooler with veggies, fruit, a six pack of bottled water and an ice pack.*
>
> *Wednesday, November 24:*
> *Alarm went off at four am. Yuck! Got into the shower, put on my favorite comfy jeans and a sweatshirt. Then I ate breakfast: one cup Kellogg's Smart Start cereal with one cup 1% milk with one banana. Loaded up the car and I was on the road by 5:00am. Driving along Interstate 5 is endless but the sunrise this morning was like a big orange sunburst hanging in the sky, at times very distracting with the big orange glaring into my eyes.*
>
> 8:00 am: *Stopped at Harris Ranch for breakfast while I waited for my sister to pick me up. This restaurant was packed with other travelers and gave the morning a festive feel. I ordered an Egg Beater omelet with mushrooms and tomatoes. No cheese. Coffee w/cream, side order of fruit which included melons and bananas. One bagel, no butter, with strawberry jelly.*

10:00 am: *Snack—energy bar.*

Noon: *Arrived at Mom's and quickly unloaded the car and went to eat: Subway Sandwich: turkey on whole wheat, mustard, lettuce, tomato, and pickles (no mayo, no cheese). One small bag of BBQ Baked Lays and a Diet Pepsi.*

2:00 pm: *Snack—baby carrots with non-fat ranch salad dressing.*

4:00 pm: *Snack—green sour apple. Very crunchy and sour! YUMMY!*

4:15 pm: *My sister and I went for a great bike ride through the Ojai valley complete with hills and a quad-burning workout. The sun was warm, about 70 degrees, and a very slight breeze. We rode about 10 miles. It felt great to get the blood moving after a long drive.*

6:00 pm: *Dinner out at a Mexican restaurant included: vegetarian burrito with grilled chicken. No cheese, no sour cream, no guacamole. Green salad, w/lemon. Non-fat yogurt for dessert.*

Thursday, November 25 THANKSGIVING DAY:

6:30 am: *Ran a tough three miles with my stepfather through his avocado orchard course. I did fine until the turnaround point, but the last hill really killed me. It was tough to keep up with him as he's a whole foot taller than I am and runs faster. It was a great workout. A super way to start Thanksgiving.*

7:30 am: *Breakfast—whole wheat bagel with two tablespoons reduced-fat crunchy peanut butter, banana, non-fat latte.*

10:00 am: *Snack—energy bar*

Noon: *Snack—banana*

2:00 pm: *Thanksgiving meal—white meat turkey, mashed potatoes, salad, dinner roll.*

5:00 pm: *Dessert at Grandma's. Half-piece pumpkin pie with whipped cream.*

Friday, November 26

7:00 am: *Four-mile run along the avocado groves. I felt like slug bait and walked the first mile to get my body used to the idea of working out. Then I ran three miles and felt good. Watching the city wake up is priceless!*

9:00 am: *Breakfast—cinnamon raisin bagel with two tablespoons reduced-fat peanut butter, banana, non-fat latte.*

Noon: *Turkey sandwich w/mustard, tomato lettuce, pickles (no mayo). BBQ baked Lays, diet Pepsi*

3:00 pm: *Fruit salad at Grandma's! Complete with strawberries, bananas and various melons.*

6:00 pm: *Dinner at Marie Callendar's restaurant. Grilled-chicken penne pasta with red sauce. Green salad with tomato vinaigrette. Half piece of no-sugar Razzleberry pie with whipped cream (split it with my sister).*

Saturday, November 27:
No workout: Scheduled rest day

7:00 am: *Breakfast—oatmeal with raisins, non-fat latte*

10:00 am: *Snack—apple*
Driving back to Northern California

Noon: *Ate lunch at roadside restaurant: Turkey salad with non-fat honey mustard dressing, with two saltine crackers.*

3:00 pm: *Snack—apple*

6:00 pm: *Arrived home—chicken noodle soup with crackers, green salad with non-fat ranch dressing.*

Sunday, November 28
10K Race in Golden Gate Park

Some final tips

I made sure to have a bottle of water with me at all times. Generally speaking, I drink tons daily! I always have energy bars or a piece of fruit with me; that way I rely on myself if I get hungry. The week was very full with visiting friends and family. With three ill relatives, I was trying to help out as much as possible. And as you may experience in a packed holiday household, it can be stressful dealing with all the various personalities. Some days I was able to handle the family stuff better than others. I'm proud to say I didn't resort to bingeing on unhealthy foods as I've done in many years past. Hopefully, with these tips you can eat healthy through the holidays too.

Fantastic Joan Salge Blake recipes

My friend and registered dietician, Joan Salge Blake, offers several great recipes for those of you that do cook (unlike me) and want some guidance. Joan creates these recipes and posts them at ThriveOnline (www.thriveonline.com), a health web site where she is the resident nutrition expert. Believe me, if I were of a mind to cook and/or prepare food, these recipes are the ones I would enjoy.

Easy Italian Meatballs

1 pound ground turkey

1 cup Italian seasoned breadcrumbs

1 egg, slightly beaten

3 cups spaghetti sauce

In a large bowl, combine ground turkey, breadcrumbs and egg until blended. Roll into 16 meatballs. Place meatballs in a single row, along the edge of a large, round, covered microwave-proof baking dish to form a complete circle. Microwave on High for 5 minutes. Turn meats over and cook on High for another 5 minutes or until the internal temperature of the meatballs reach at least 165°F when measured with a meat thermometer. *Note: This is based on a 850 watt microwave oven. Microwave ovens differ so check your instruction manual for the proper length of cooking time.* In a large pot, heat spaghetti sauce until bubbly hot. Add hot meatballs to sauce and serve. Makes 16 meatballs.

PER MEATBALL:
CALORIES: 114   *FAT:* 5.5 G   *SATURATED FAT:* 1 G   *CHOLESTEROL:* 34 MG   *SODIUM:* 342 MG   *FIBER:* 1 G

CREATED BY JOAN SALGE BLAKE, MS, RD

Grilled Veggie Pizza

1 large red pepper, sliced into 1 inch slices

2 cups raw broccoli florets

1 raw onion, sliced

8 ounces, pre-sliced portabella mushrooms

6 Tbls light Sweet Vidalia Onion Salad Dressing or Light Creamy Italian Salad Dressing

1/3 cup tomato sauce or spaghetti sauce

1 cup shredded part skim mozzarella cheese

4 Tbls shredded Parmesan cheese

1 Italian-style flatbread pizza shell

Preheat 425°F oven. Place shell on baking sheet and set aside. Brush veggies with salad dressing and grill, broil, or stir fry under tender. Remove veggies from grill and place clean plate or dish. Spread spaghetti sauce even over pizza. Sprinkle with mozzarella cheese. Top with grilled vegetables and then Parmesan cheese. Bake for 10 to 12 minutes or until pizza is hot and bubbly. Serves 8.

PER SERVING:
CALORIES: 243   *FAT:* 6 G   *SATURATED FAT:* 1.5 G   *CHOLESTEROL:* 0 MG   *SODIUM:* 473 MG   *FIBER:* 2 G

CREATED BY JOAN SALGE BLAKE, MS, RD

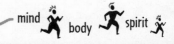

mind body spirit

Seasoned Roasted Red Potatoes

> 2 pounds small red potatoes, washed
>
> 1 1/2 tsp olive oil
>
> 1/2 tsp Italian seasoning
>
> 3 tbls Parmesan cheese
>
> vegetable oil spray

Preheat oven to 375°F. Slice potatoes into quarters and place in large bowl. Drizzle with olive oil and toss. Spray baking sheet with vegetable oil spray. Place potatoes on sheet and sprinkle with seasoning and cheese. Bake for 55 minutes or until golden brown. Makes 8 servings.

PER SERVING:
CALORIES: 185   FAT: 1.5 G   SATURATED FAT: 0.5 G   CHOLESTEROL: 2 MG   SODIUM: 57 MG

CREATED BY JOAN SALGE BLAKE, MS, RD

Spinach Stuffed Spuds

> 4 baking potatoes, about 2 1/2 pounds
>
> 10 oz package chopped spinach, thawed
>
> 3 tbls light margarine
>
> 1 cup chopped onions
>
> 2 tbls skim milk
>
> 6 ounces light sharp cheddar cheese, shredded
>
> 1/4 tsp salt
>
> 1/8 tsp pepper

Preheat oven to 425°F. Wash and scrub potatoes. Pierce skins with fork. Bake for 45 minutes to one hour until done. Set aside. Reduce oven heat to 350°F. Place spinach in a colander and squeeze out excess water. Place spinach in bowl. Slice potatoes length-wise in half. Carefully scoop out inside of potato, leaving skin and approximately 1/4 inch rim of potato. Add the scooped out potato to spinach in bowl. Sauté onions in one tablespoon margarine until tender. Add to spinach mixture along with milk, four ounces of cheese, salt, and pepper. Blend. Scoop mixture evenly into potato skins. Bake for 15 to 20 minutes or until hot. Top with remaining cheese and continue baking for about 3 minutes or until cheese is melted. Makes 8 stuffed potatoes.

EACH STUFFED POTATO:
CALORIES: 302   FAT: 6 G   SATURATED FAT: 2.5 G   CHOLESTEROL: 15 MG   SODIUM: 295 MG

CREATED BY JOAN SALGE BLAKE, MS, RD

Carrot Raisin Bread

1 1/2 cup whole wheat flour 1 egg, beaten

1/4 cup plus 2 tbls sugar

2 tsp baking powder

1/4 tsp baking soda

1 1/2 tsp ground cinnamon

1/2 tsp allspice

1/2 cup water

1 tbls oil

1/2 tsp vanilla

12 ounce baby food carrots

3/4 cup raisins

Preheat oven to 350°F. Lightly oil loaf pan. Stir together dry ingredients. In separate bowl, mix together remaining ingredients; add this mixture to dry mixture. Stir to moisten. Spoon into baking pan. Bake 50 minutes or until toothpick inserted in center comes out clean. Cool 5 minute in pan. Invert on wire rack for continued cooling. Makes 16 slices.

PER SERVING:
CALORIES: 94   *FAT:* 1.5 G   *CHOLESTEROL:* 13 MG   *SODIUM:* 68 MG   *FIBER:* 2 G

CREATED BY JOAN SALGE BLAKE, MS, RD

mind   body   spirit

Pumpkin Cheesecake Pie

For the crust:

>   1 cup oatmeal
>
>   1 1/2 tsp tub style margarine
>
>   1/2 cup honey crunch-style wheat germ
>
>   3 tbls brown sugar
>
>   1 egg white

For the pie:

>   1 cup low fat cottage cheese
>
>   4 ounces cream cheese, 1/3 less fat neufchatel
>
>   1/2 cup sugar
>
>   1/2 cup canned pumpkin
>
>   3 tbls flour
>
>   1 tsp vanilla
>
>   1 tsp pumpkin spice
>
>   2 egg whites

Preheat oven to 325°F. Spray a 9-inch pie pan with vegetable oil spray. Set aside. In non-stick fry pan, melt margarine. Add oatmeal and toast until slightly golden, approximately 2 minutes. Remove from heat and spoon oatmeal into a small bowl. Add wheat germ, brown sugar, and egg white. Mix until crumbly. Pat into the bottom and sides of the pie pan. Set aside. In blender or food processor, puree together all remaining ingredients except for egg whites. Blend until smooth. Pour into large bowl. Slightly beat egg whites with a fork and gently fold into mixture. Pour mixture into pie pan and bake for 50 minutes or until center of cheesecake is firm. Makes 8 servings.

PER SERVING:
CALORIES: 219   *FAT:* 6   *SATURATED FAT:* 2.5 G   *CHOLESTEROL:* 14 MG   *SODIUM:* 206 MG   *FIBER:* 0.5 G

CREATED BY JOAN SALGE BLAKE, MS, RD

Pumpkin Date Nut Muffins

1 cup bran cereal (nugget-type)

1 cup apple juice

1 1/2 cup whole wheat flour

1 tbls baking powder

1/2 cup brown sugar, packed

1 tsp pumpkin pie spice

1/4 cup chopped walnuts

1 tbls vegetable oil

2 egg whites

1 cup canned pumpkin

1 cup chopped dates

Preheat oven to 400°F. In a small mixing bowl, combine bran cereal and apple juice. Let stand. In a large mixing bowl, combine flour, baking powder, brown sugar, pumpkin pie spice, and walnuts. Stir to blend. Add oil, egg whites, and pumpkin to cereal mixture. Stir until well blended. Add cereal mixture to large mixing bowl. Stir until just blended. Add dates and stir. Spoon muffin mixture into 12 muffin tins that have been coated with vegetable oil spray. Bake for 18 minutes or until toothpick inserted in center is clean when removed. Makes 12 muffins.

PER MUFFIN:
CALORIES: 180   *FAT:* 3.5 G   *SATURATED FAT:* <0.5 G   *SODIUM:* 58 MG   *CHOLESTEROL:* 0 MG   *DIETARY FIBER:* 5.5 G

CREATED BY JOAN SALGE BLAKE, MS, RD

mind body spirit

FOOD 101 plan

Food is one of those things that we can't avoid. We simply have to eat. So, if food has been a challenge like it has for me all my life, you need a plan. You need some guidance on how to deal with food. Here are some things for you to remember in making your own plan to come to terms with food in your life.

1 **Diets don't work.** Accept the fact that starving yourself from time to time in an effort to lose weight never works in the long run. You must eat, even if you're fat.

2 **Eat lower in fat, lower in sugar, high in fiber, and variety.** Cut back on the junk and go for a balanced diet. You've heard it before: fruits and vegetables, lean meats, low fat dairy, and whole grains.

3 **Eat little meals or snacks throughout the day.** This should give you energy throughout the day and avoid hunger.

4 **Drink lots of water every day.** Ideally, drink at least eight glasses or 64 ounces of water or non-caffeinated fluids per day. Remember your fluid needs increase with exercise.

5 **Log what you eat.** To avoid overeating, this is one way to keep things in check for yourself. Write out everything in log or notebook. I use a software program called Lifeform (www.lifeform.com).

6 **Limit alcohol.** Alcohol can be dehydrating and add calories to your diet.

7 **Be realistic.** This is important especially when you first start out attempting to correct your eating habits. For example, it is next to impossible to just cold turkey your fast food eating habit. Deciding one day that you will never have another huge cheeseburger and large fries is not realistic. It is more realistic to gradually cut back on the less healthy stuff from your menu. Weaning yourself from fatty foods is going to be very difficult. It is okay to occasionally have a burger or a pepperoni pizza, just try not to make it a daily habit. I know of a long distance runner who allows himself one cheeseburger a week, so I know it's possible to eat that but not go crazy!

Staying committed

I don't see the sense in any of this. I was out walking trying to get my health back on track and this is the thanks I get. It's so frustrating when things don't seem to be fair. I know there's probably a good reason for all of this, but damn if any of it makes sense to me now. I'm trying to eat healthy and watch my portions since I'm not able to workout while recovering. I took my exercise time for granted. I complained and whined about it all the time and now I can't wait to get out there and appreciate what my body can do for me. Never again will I take my health for granted. I know I'm impatient with myself. Perhaps that's the lesson in all of this? Who knows?

JOURNAL ENTRY, MARCH 17, 1997

There probably isn't a person alive today that doesn't know how important it is to be active and make good food choices. So how come dropout rates for people who start an exercise routine are 50 percent or greater by the end of a six month period? I would bet that it's not because these people don't know how beneficial a lifestyle change is, but because it's hard as hell to stay committed to fitness and health even when you have been doing it for a while.

So what is it that makes us miss days, lose enthusiasm, etc.? I would say that at least three different aspects of working out affect your desire to continue on a long-term basis: you, the workout itself, and your workout environment.

Practical issues
It's your body!

You made the choice weeks, months or even years ago to change your lifestyle. Your focus is solid, but there are days that you just don't make it to the gym, out the door, or on to the stationary bike. This has everything to do with your feelings about exercise. Maybe in your life exercise has always represented something of a grind, an onerous task that leaves you with a bad taste or just plain sick of it. Maybe you can't get past that feeling of walking into a gym filled with "beautiful bodies." Maybe you need something to hone your discipline level, even though you may have been exercising consistently until now.

mind 🏃 body 🏃 spirit 🏃

Working out is about making a physical *and* a mental course change. If you are still self-conscious at the gym, try a new place or exercise outside or on a treadmill at home. If you are stuck in the "I've tried this before and failed miserably" phase, picture (literally) a beautiful new leaf turning over—that is what you are doing for your body when you work out. If you are struggling with discipline—and even the most conditioned athletes do at some point—try keeping a journal or a workout log. Having your accomplishments on paper (or on the computer) can do wonders for your motivation (who wants a "zero" on their log, right?).

I NEVER was an early riser, but after a few weeks of JUST DOING IT! It became a way of life! I now can go to a gym after I drop my daughter off at school, but I have to just go straight there or I could start looking for excuses! The eating healthy is ALWAYS going to be tough, but I look at OLD photos (I carry one in my purse of me at 250) and say NO WAY can I go back to that life, and mostly I look at my beautiful 5 year old daughter Kenzie and think if I go back to that life I might not live to see her be SUCCESSFUL in her life!   LYNNELL, CONNECTING IN FL

When you've run through all the traditional ways of staying motivated, then is the time to pour on the "no more excuses" determination. Like a second wind that you get (if you're lucky) while running, that determination allows you to pull energy from within and get stuff done. I think being determined, actually talking to yourself about it if you have to, is what makes your exercise a lifestyle change and not just a pastime.

And let's not get crazy here. While you are changing your mental programming, you don't have to go over the deep end to where it's all you think about. Strive for balance. If working out four or five days a week is what works for you right now, then that's great! Taking a few days off during the week is healthy and can be the break that your body needs to really perform the next time. It's also "head healthy" because you're not punishing yourself for not doing something that day.

A new adventure

The next thing that could have your motivation dragging in the mud is the rut you've gotten into with your workouts. Are you doing the same run five times a week? Or are you walking in circles around a track because it's safer than being on the street? Is your workout at a convenient time of the day?

Are you pushing yourself so hard that it's not fun anymore? These and many other sinkholes are not uncommon. It's in our very human nature to do something to death, and believe it or not, we all need change once in a while!

If you have always worked out inside, try buying a map of nearby nature trails or state parks within easy driving distance. The change of scenery will lift a heavy mental load. Vary your workout. If you are running the same five miles each day, mix in some speed work or even some fast walking. Better yet, get up early, pack a lunch and go for a brisk hike with someone you love. At an advanced fitness level, you can even try things that you never thought were possible, like taking a rock-climbing class (start on an indoor wall or outside). If you're not already, substitute a few days a week of your regular workout with some cross-training activity, like mountain biking, weight-lifting or jumping rope.

Of course, my favorite advice when things get stale is (you should know this by heart by now) set a goal! Not only does this help your focus and motivation, but you really challenge yourself. It doesn't have to be a competition. It can be a long hiking trip through Europe or an afternoon spent mountain biking.

Although this isn't a necessity, I think it can be fun to check out health expos. One of the neatest things is seeing the newest in clothing and gadgets. Sometimes a new gadget to keep track of your exercise time or heart rate, the newest in high tech clothing or just being surrounded by other people who are as interested in their health and fitness as you are can give you a real lift.

My watch motivator

These days the most impressive watches for running are on the market. Nike, Speedo, Adidas, and several other athletic firms make them to not only keep time, but to monitor the number of laps you do around a track, and to check on your speed for each lap. The real fancy watches will even tell you how many miles you have gone.

Quick Reference Checklist for Motivation

· Baby steps! Progress one small goal at a time

· Find someone you can look up to if you need to; having a mentor can be really inspirational

· Keep a journal—this is a great place to air your feelings and chart your progress

· Set up a reward system to keep yourself motivated to work out

· Vary your workouts to keep them a "get to" and not a "have to" part of your life

· Information can be a powerful tool; read fitness and motivational books to keep your mental focus

· Concentrate on being able to do *more* things you never thought you could

mind body spirit

For me, I use a watch when I run on a track as a way to improve the time to do a lap. This keeps me motivated and keeps my workout interesting. I compete with myself and the watch. I think: "Okay, last time it took me such-an-so minutes to do a lap, this time I will try to better myself by half a minute." Or whatever. The idea is to use a watch, a lap counter, a pedometer, a radio, or whatever it takes to keep you going.

A little help from my friends

Your surroundings can have a huge effect on your motivation to work out. So can *who* you work out with. Although I personally work out by myself because it's such a good time for me to think and have solitude, I like running with people, too. Fitness buddies can add a light, social element to your workout and lift you out of a motivation rut. Asking a friend who has a similar focus on fitness to be your workout partner can help you get your butt out of bed in the morning—especially if you know he or she is waiting for you. You can find fitness buddies online or find a walking or running club in your city.

Mental issues
Struggle

It was Frederick Douglass who said, "if there is not struggle, there is no progress." If you're out living life and participating in life, you will have struggles. Just part of this whole thing. I have struggles everyday. Things I need to sort through. I guess my attitude has changed toward these struggles. I know as long as I resist, the problem will persist.

I still have a ways to go as far as the weight is concerned but the most amazing change is that the weight doesn't even matter as much. Funny how the thing that was constantly troubling me for years is now not such a big deal. I am out there in shorts and a tank top running and I don't even think about it! I know I'm on the right track and the weight will take care of itself.   CAROL, CONNECTING IN IA

So, now what I try and do is just let my mind "sort through it all" I don't put pressure on myself that I have to figure everything out. I just keep asking powerful questions. Reminding myself what my priorities are and what my goals are and how I can keep moving toward my goals etc. Some days it feels like I'm going backwards, and, let's face it some days I am. But I don't quit. And the very next opportunity I get, I put one foot in front of the other and press on.

Cut yourself some slack! I give you all permission! You don't need to solve everything *today*. Be open to the sorting out process. It's all part of the journey. As long as you keep open minded and ask yourself powerful questions on how you can learn and get through this time a better person, and not bitter, you'll enjoy the process. What's happened to me is that I don't get as frustrated as I used to. I still have frustrations. Hey, I'm human. But it's not at the level that I used to suffer.

Remember pain is inevitable; suffering is optional.

Fans & detractors

When you leave your old life behind, you'll inevitably leave some of the people and things in your old life behind, too. I had friends, all over 200 pounds, who seemed supportive before I started losing all my weight through exercise, but now they say I've lost too much weight. It went farther than that. A few months ago, they got together and did an *intervention* because they were so "concerned" about my lifestyle changes. I heard things like, "You're completely obsessed with weight," "You're too thin," "You need counseling," etc. Obviously this didn't do much for our friendship.

So my lesson from all that is look within yourself. Surround yourself with people who are living the lifestyle you do. Because things that used to be acceptable won't be acceptable anymore. For instance, eating at night. People would ask me out to dinner and wouldn't want to eat until 8 or 9 at night and I was training for a marathon and I would say, no, I can't stay out that late. If you want to eat at 6, I'll meet you there and I'd love to see you, but my workouts are a priority and these are the choices that I have to make.

It is not uncommon for spouses, or siblings, or parents, or friends (even best friends), co-workers, and others to find it difficult to accept the fact that you are a new person. They are used to the old you, they may not like the idea that you are committed to losing weight, engaging in healthy activ-

· More than 60 percent of U.S. women do not engage in the recommended amount of physical activity.

· More than 25 percent of U.S. women are not active at all.

· Physical inactivity is more common among women than men.

· Social support from family and friends has been consistently and positively related to regular physical activity.

CENTERS FOR DISEASE CONTROL, NATIONAL CENTER FOR CHRONIC DISEASE PREVENTION AND HEALTH PROMOTION, PHYSICAL ACTIVITY AND HEALTH REPORT, 11/99

mind 🏃 body 🏃 spirit 🏃

ities like exercise, not smoking, not drinking, not eating pizzas and cheese-burgers with reckless abandon, and so on.

Unfortunately, I must tell you to expect criticism, rude comments, sarcasm, and other discouraging things. You may even have to prepare yourself for rejection. Keep in mind, by changing, this can intimidate and possibly instill feelings of jealousy or envy in people you least expect to treat you this way. It is odd, you might think, as I once did that your friends and family, people close to you, would be supportive. Logically, rationally, you might think they want you to become healthy and happy. And yet, they can turn out to be the very ones who are least likely to give you the support you need.

For me, the response was mixed. Some of my friends, as I just mentioned, thought I had gone off the deep end. They thought I had become obsessed. My sister is very much impressed by the changes I have made. And Martin, thank goodness, has stuck with me throughout, offering ongoing encouragement and celebrating my successes.

Certain family members think I'm nuts for quitting a "perfect" corporate sales job to write this book and work on the Connectors web site full time. There was a time in my life when this lack of support would have given me a perfect excuse for quitting. Not anymore. I am much more of an independent person now than I was when I was working at playing the victim full time. It would be wonderful to have their approval, but I know that I can't base my life and my decisions on what they think. I look for approval now on my own terms, instead of seeking it from people who cannot give it to me.

What is important is to know that you are doing the right thing for yourself. Fortunately, I have the support and offer support to the Connectors who I share my experience with every day online. And it is greatly inspiring and encouraging to learn about their experiences and to meet with them at the races where we get together. This is what helps keep going. Besides, I know I just can't go back to where I was.

I am an athlete. I am a marathoner. I love to run. I never thought I would use these sentences to describe myself. My lifelong battle with weight began when I was just a child. For much of my life, I gained and lost, gained and lost. My brain turned fat too, destroying my self-esteem.

A couple of years ago I decided to start working out again. Last year, I decided to run a marathon. I hated running, so I signed up for a marathon training club. The first time I ran with the group, I made it about 1/2 mile and I cried. I wanted to give up. At that moment, I thought I was crazy for even attempting a marathon. My fat brain was taking over again. About two months before the marathon, I decided to stop saying that I hate to run. Instead I started chanting "I love to run" as I trotted along. Amazingly enough, it worked. It became my mantra when the going got tough on long runs.

During one of my training runs, a Pit bull dog attacked me. No permanent damage was done…physically. Shortly after that, a man purposely threw his lit cigarette at me from his car. I kept running. All of the sudden it clicked. My fat brain didn't stop me! I KEPT RUNNING! After all by this time, I loved to run.

When I got home that day, after taking a shower, I looked at myself in the mirror and saw the most beautiful woman staring back at me. A transformation had taken place over the past two years…my fat brain went into recession. Still present, but not as dominating as my skinny brain. I realized that my fat brain was holding me back and it had been holding me back from reaching my potential for the better part of 22 years
KIRSTEN, CONNECTING IN CA

Doubt

Life doesn't always make sense. For instance, I have days where I think, I have lost a lot of weight and I really do feel much better physically and mentally. My body fat is down and I finally am at the point where I feel like I look fine. But the other side of the coin is that I work out six days a week—running, weights, water fitness—and I eat healthy, and yet I still have rolls of fat on me when I sit down. I feel like stamping my foot on the ground and yelling, "it's not fair! I have been at this for three years and I still am not at goal weight!" Never mind that I don't even know what goal weight is most of the time because I am so busy taking things one day at a time.

Other things nag me, too. Here I am leading a huge group of people and that makes me feel internal pressure just because of the way I am naturally. It's in my nature to want things to be perfect—and they aren't. I have this feeling that I am supposed to have all the answers and, surprise! I don't! I don't know why I am not at this mythical "goal weight." I even catch myself falling into the typical trap of wanting to lose weight really fast—that instant gratification, get it over with now instinct.

mind 🏃 body 🏃 spirit 🏃

So, what do I do when I doubt my lifestyle choices? First of all, I take a deep breath and remind myself that I am just a regular person with the same daily frustrations as everyone else. I have to wait in line at the post office, the grocery store, and the bank. I tell myself that even if the doubt *never* completely disappears (and it probably won't), I have still come a long and wonderful way from where I was.

If I use butter on my toast, if I go back to eating creamy sauces on my pasta, using the elevator instead of the stairs, or sleep instead of getting up and moving, I will spend the rest of my life, waiting for tomorrow before I change my life. Plus, all of the changes that I have made over the past 18 months will have been wasted.

NANCY, CONNECTING IN TN

If you have doubts that creep into your head and try to make you think you're crazy for doing what you're doing, just stop and ask yourself to name two or three things that are better now than they were a year ago, a month ago, a day ago. Maybe today you were able to get to that gallon of water. Or a month ago you couldn't run at all and now you are running two miles. Whatever it is, you need to confirm the positive and the strides you have made.

Frustration

Hello common occurrence! It seems that there is always something to be frustrated by, least of all our health and fitness progress. So, how do you deal with the frustration?

- I always have goals that I am working toward, whether they are big or small. If I didn't have goals that were important to me that I could pursue and it was just about losing weight, I would have quit a long time ago.

- Let's resolve the myth of what is "fair" in life. In fact, let's throw the whole notion out. Why? Because asking "what should I expect?" or "what will be fair for me?" is like saying, get out the crystal ball and tell me what the future holds. *You* hold the future. Your choices today *make* the future you have tomorrow.

  So is it fair that you work out five or six days a week and not immediately see anything come of it or that the results are slower than you want? Maybe in the traditional sense of the word, no. But in the sense that every positive step that you take for yourself is a step forward, yes, it's fair. "It's not fair" is what you say when you don't know what you will do the next day.

- Life throws us many curveballs and we have to learn to adapt and stay focused. People will try to knock you off your course, for whatever reason, or things will come up that try to pull us off the track we are on, so if your focus is steady, you will be able to prevail. It's sort of the make lemonade from lemons idea.

Physical plateaus

It's easy to become frustrated by arriving at a plateau in your fitness program where you are at a standstill weight-wise or goal-wise. This is a very common problem, but that doesn't make it any easier to deal with in terms of losing your desire to continue your fitness routine. Ask yourself, are my goals realistic? Have I set small enough goals on the way to my overall goal that I can actually make progress? Be aware, too, that making a physical change in your body can take at least a month, depending on the physical condition you are in when you start. All of us want a "quick fix," but we know deep down there's no such thing.

It helps to understand how your body reacts to the new exercise routine you are undergoing. In the first four weeks, your training is mostly about your body learning how to use your muscles and increase strength. That's why it's important to take your emphasis off of weight—while you may lose fat weight, remember, muscle weighs more than fat, so you may be under the impression that you are actually *gaining* weight at first. The great thing is that as you add muscle, you actually are progressing forward in a positive way since muscle speeds your metabolism and burns calories more efficiently. Measure your success in more relevant ways: how do you feel about yourself since you started working out? Do you have more energy? How do your clothes fit?

I was 35 pounds overweight and could barely squeeze into pants that are a size I don't want to think about, much less admit; and then I hear someone complaining about not being able to lose five or ten pounds. I find myself thinking, "Oh, PUHLEEZE—Give me a break! If I was only 10 pounds from goal I'd lose that weight so fast it would make your head spin! Do you know how many times I've lost 10 pounds? Hundreds! I'm an expert at losing 10 pounds. Do you know how lucky you are? What's your problem that you can't lose a measly ol' 10 pounds?"

mind   body   spirit

Well, then it was my turn to be 10 pounds from goal. I worked hard to change my lifestyle and lose the first 25 pounds. And then all of a sudden things came to a grinding halt. What seemed to work before now didn't have the same effect. Welcome to the danger zone. Food that I'd left behind reared its head and said, "Remember me and how great I tasted?" Getting up at 5am to work out became a struggle after 5 months of daily exercise without a second thought. I was able to wear some of my 'thin' clothes, and began to ask myself why I should take on the extra effort. I could either get complacent and fall into the seductive trap I have countless times before and let go of my commitment to living a healthier life, or I could crank things up a notch.

Thanks to Tawni and other Connectors I was able to choose the latter and can gratefully say that those remaining 10 pounds are gone and have stayed gone. I decided to do three things:

1. I admitted to my fellow Connectors that I was on a slippery slope. (Of all the action steps, this was the hardest for my pride to handle.)

2. I wrote Tawni and asked if I could hire her as a coach so I could benefit from her motivation and determination, while I lost this last 10 pounds.

3. I wrote what I was feeling in a journal and went on a search to discover the reasons behind my self-destructive behavior.

Here is what happened as a result of those three actions:

1. The Connectors were absolutely supportive. There were no judgments and they suggested I check in more regularly during this tougher time. One even sent me her phone number to call if necessary, and others cheered me on, expressing their faith in my ability to overcome this challenge. If I had been left to myself I'd have mentally beaten myself up over the weight gain and probably resorted to 'comfort' food to ease the frustration. Knowing that I wasn't alone helped motivate me to get back on track.

2. Being accountable to Tawni, who had come so much farther than I was even attempting, was a powerful experience. I emailed her daily and received prompt replies, full of specific encouragement. When we spoke on the phone each week she was very attentive and did not skirt around tough questions as we were looking at what I was living.

3. I got a new spiral binder and started writing. I first described what had been going on and asked myself why I was starting to abandon menus that were plentiful with items I enjoyed and had been perfectly sufficient up until I hit the "10 pounds to goal" mark.

Tawni talks about the spirit of the Connectors. It is this spirit that supplied the extra boost that made this weight loss the last weight loss; and for the first time provided an impetus for a healthy and fit life, instead of a continual longing for a thinner, healthier someday in the future. NATASHA, CONNECTING IN WY

Go online & get help!

I cannot say enough about how the Connectors have helped me maintain my motivation, even during times of stress. Nothing can replace that reaching out spirit and mutual support because everyone is either going through it, too or someone has been there and will tell you how to get through it. If you find you're struggling with staying motivated and on track, join forces with another Connector! It works! We're our own best defense.

Whenever I meet up with some local Connectors, I love seeing all their progress. Each month when we meet up, I see a little more confidence and pride. When was the last time you were *proud* of yourself? I think that as adults we often lose sight of what is important personally. Do we do things in our lives that make us proud? Do we keep the bar raised high, or settle on a constant basis? Well, I don't know about the rest of you, but I settled for a lot less in my twenties and I like it better keeping that bar raised high. Going for it really is a rush! Try it sometime!

Staying motivated to reach my goals

Goals help me stay motivated. I know many of you refuse to believe the POWER in setting goals, but it really does work. If I never set goals I would have quit this exercise stuff a long time ago. It's not like the weight falls off of me. So, if I was doing this exercise stuff to lose weight, it would have lost its luster after about a month, maybe two. But, with fitness goals written down, it's much easier for me to crawl out of bed.

I only write down the goals I really want. Otherwise I know I won't make the effort and sacrifices needed to get there. I have goals for all aspects of my life, so weight loss and exercise are not my only focus. There's a whole world of opportunities out there for us to pursue.

Remember none of this is done overnight. Take it one step at a time. Just don't give up. When you're having a really awful day, reach out to somebody else. It's guaranteed to make you feel better. Works for me!

mind body spirit

Fear of failure

One of the biggest reasons for fearing failure is allowing excuses to get in the way of your training. Feeling like a failure is just another way to avoid going forward. Or, another excuse to feel bad and unworthy. Then, you can beat yourself up some more, etc. SO that won't fly here! Pick yourself up, dust yourself off, and *regroup*. Make sure the goals that you set are for *you*. Be quiet and really think about what you want and how your workout routine is like many other experiences in your life. Use that experience to break through the walls of fear and failure that you've let build up in the past!

Secrets to staying committed

Here are some ways I want to share with you on how to remain committed to a lifetime of health and fitness:

1 **Avoid a rut.** Keep your routine interesting. If you run a certain course, change it at least once a week, perhaps in another location. Or cross-train with a different type of activity.

2 **Find a workout buddy.** You friends and family may not be particularly supportive, but you can find other people who are serious about health and fitness. Try local running/walking clubs, meet Connectors in your area, find out about fitness groups at specialty fitness stores, etc. A workout buddy can help keep you motivated.

3 **Post the NO MORE EXCUSES Quick Reference Motivation checklist.** Post this is in some conspicuous place in your home where you won't miss it. This is great list: finding a mentor, journaling, rewards, keeping yourself informed, trying new things, etc.

4 **Set goals.** I said it before, but I am just repeating myself here for emphasis. Goals, even the little baby steps you take, all add up. To ensure you commit yourself and achieve your goals, it is best to write them down somewhere were you can check them, daily if necessary.

5 **Don't over do it.** It is not uncommon to try too hard to achieve your goals. Take it easy. Keep things in balance. Over doing it now will only result in frustration and discourage you from continuing for the long haul.

6 **Connect with Connectors.** To make a connection with Connectors in your area can be a tremendous motivator. You can check in with them conveniently and without a whole lot of fuss. That's what is beautiful about email, you can send a message to anyone, at anytime, whether they are busy or not. You don't disturb anyone, and everyone benefits.

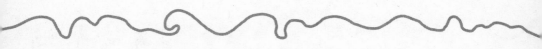

If for no other reason, this is one of the great blessings of the Internet. If you don't have a computer yet, you can go to cybercafes (coffee shops with rentable computers to go online) in nearly every major city.

About 5 years ago, I had this dream. I was a guest in a comfortable, nurturing, vibrant house in the woods where a family of women lived. I wanted to stay and live there with them. I asked to stay, and the women said (lovingly), "No, you're not ready. You still try too hard." I woke up and knew that I had best remember this dream.

I think in my life I have tried too hard because it was the only way I knew. I was banging my head against the wall, but it opened doors and I got to go places. I could ignore things and people and still make it through because I haw a big internal imagination that keeps me going in difficult times, and my capacity for denial can keep me ignorant of the price I am paying.

But now I want to go somewhere different. I want my body to truly be my home and my vehicle in life. I believe, surprisingly, that I'm changing, slowly. To change outside, i.e. lose weight, I'm changing inside, my spirit. I can't force this. I'm listening to the Connectors, and not over-training so I'm not injured. I listen to the Connectors and eat vegetables and don't eat chocolate doughnuts. I listen to my body and do what "I" tell me to do: run, run a little faster, don't run, swim instead, walk, climb. I'm holding my head a little higher, looking a few more people in the eye, feeling more open to people because I feel more authentic. The best kernel of me that's been buried inside is peeking out. I see glimpses of the wisdom of the big picture. DEBRA, CONNECTING IN CA

The one thought I want to leave you with is that the power to change your life is inside you—even if you don't feel very powerful right now. You gain power and you gain self-esteem bit by bit as you work to develop them. Just as weak muscles can be strengthened over time, a weak mental attitude can be made strong too. And if that idea seems overwhelming, focus first on the steps instead of the end result. Throughout this book I've given you lots of different lists that are really just the baby steps you take toward your goal. Focus on these steps and you'll be amazed at how your inner strength grows and takes over. The journey is exhilarating, believe me, and it begins with one simple, but heartfelt, phrase, "No more excuses!"

mind 🏃 body 🏃 spirit 🏃

Products

Active Body Exercise Clothing/Active Wear
www.primenet.com/~apfc
Great for workout clothes, swim, and casual clothing; they also have
plus sizes and major labels

Athleta: Where Women Gear Up (catalog)
888-322-5515
www.athleta.com

Contour Pak
800-926-2228
www.countourpak.com
Ice packs for injuries

Electra Sports
www.electrasports.com
877-432-7475
More than just a catalog; great info about women's health and fitness

The Greater Salt Lake Clothing Company
www.gslcc.com
801-273-8700
Plus sizes on outdoor sports and athletic wear

Hummingbird Activewear
www.hummingbirdwear.com
877-486-9327
Workout/fitness clothing; proceeds from sales go to women's disease research

Junonia
www.junonia.com
800-671-0175
A catalog for women sizes 14 and up; workout wear

Polar Heart Rate Monitors
www.pursuit-performance.com.au

Precor
www.precor.com
Makers of home/commercial exercise equipment; they are top of the line

Roadrunner Sports
800-551-5558
www.roadrunnersports.com

SportHill (catalog)
800-622-8444
Good for larger sizes

The Sports Basement
415-437-0100 ext. 5
www.sportsbasement.com
Closeout brand name sports wear

Title Nine Sports: A Catalog Inspired by and Created for Women
800-609-0092

Tunturi
www.tunturi.com
Makers of high quality, reasonably priced indoor fitness equipment

Books

Runner's World Complete Book of Running: Everything You Need to Know to Run for Fun, Fitness, and Competition.
Burfoot, Amby, editor, Emmaus, PA: Rodale Press, Inc., 1997.
An excellent overview of a variety of aspects of running, mental and physical.

Bailey, Covert & Gates, Ronda. *Smart Eating: Choosing Wisely, Living Lean.*
New York, NY: Houghton Mifflin, 1996.
A great place to re-learn how to eat; excellent recipes, too.

Bailey, Covert. *The New Fit or Fat.*
New York, NY: Houghton Mifflin, 1991.
One of the best primers ever written on being fit.

Breathnach, Sarah Ban. Simple Abundance Journal of Gratitude.
New York: Warner Books, 1996.
I love this because it's so nicely laid out and gives me plenty to be thankful for.

Galloway, Jeff. *Marathon!*
Phidippides Publishing, 1996.
The book that convinced me I could run a marathon.

Kersey, Cynthia. *Unstoppable.*
Naperville, IL: Sourcebooks, Inc., 1998.
Great inspiring stories of perseverance and triumph.

Kortge, Carolyn Scott. *The Spirited Walker: Fitness Walking for Clarity, Balance, and Spiritual Connection.*
San Francisco, CA: Harper Collins, 1998.
Takes walking to another level.

McGraw, Phillip. Life Strategies: Doing What Works, Doing What Matters.
New York: Hyperion, 1999.
Much of what this book says rings so true inside me.

Pipher, Mary, PhD. *Reviving Ophelia: Saving the Selves of Adolescent Girls.*
New York, NY: Ballantine, 1994.
Fascinating look at how girls are influenced in their childhood.

Sheehan, Dr. George. *Running & Being: The Total Experience.*
Red Bank, NJ: Second Wind, 1978.
The ultimate runner's philosopher talks about running and life.

Zukav, Gary. The Seat of the Soul.
New York: Fireside Books, 1990.
Very inspiring.

Magazines

Runner's World magazine
Customer service/subscriptions: 800-666-2828
Or write to: Runner's World Magazine
                      PO Box 7307
                      Red Oak, IA 51591

Or check out their web site:
www.runnersworld.com

Walking Magazine
Customer service/subscriptions: 800-248-6827
Or write to: Walking Magazine
                      Reader's Digest Association, Inc.
                      7501 Winstead Drive
                      Louisville, Kentucky 40281-2222

Or check out their web site:
www.walkingmag.com

Web sites

American Health for Women
www.americanhealth.com

Living Fit (Fitness Online)
www.livingfit.com
Very informative fitness, health and nutrition site

ThriveOnline
www.thriveonline.com
or on AOL, keyword: Thrive

The Water Dance web site
www.waterdanceonline.com
Info about water fitness

SPECIAL ACKNOWLEDGEMENT

I wish to thank two special consultants who have helped me make this a better book. I wish to thank Dr. Amy Roberts and Joan Salge Blake for their expertise in fitness and nutrition, respectively.

Dr. Amy Roberts

Dr. Amy Roberts helped me smooth out my writing about and clarify my understanding of fitness. Amy is based out of the Boulder Center for Sports Medicine and is an established expert in cardiovascular fitness and athletic performance. She is an advisor for the Colorado Avalanche, Denver Nuggets, U.S. Cycling team, U.S. Cross Country Ski Team, and a number of other professional and elite athletes. She holds a Masters and Doctorate in Physiology from the University of California at Berkeley and is a fellow in the American College of Sports Medicine. Amy also sits on the boards of both the Boulder Chapter of the American Heart Association and the Rocky Mountain Chapter of the American College of Sports Medicine. Her work is regularly published and reviewed in peer journals around the country.

Believe it or not, this academic finds some time for fun, too. Amy's friends tell her she excels at sports that keep her moving in a straight line. But she is also working to expand her activity portfolio to include sports that actually require some hand-eye coordination. Amy loves to run, ski, and bike. And lately she's been trying her hand, so to speak, at rock climbing and ultimate Frisbee.

And yes, that would be the same Amy you saw playing in the symphony and swing-dancing at the local bar. In addition, she's a fan of funky tunes, blues, and good wine.

Joan Salge Blake

Joan Salge Blake, MS, RD, is a nutrition consultant who has done much to improve my discussion on food and nutrition in Food 101. She has also provided some excellent high nutrition, low fat recipes. Joan is a regular consultant for ThriveOnline, the popular health/fitness and nutrition web site.

Joan grew up in a noisy Italian family in New Jersey. (She was a cheerleader in high school, which may explain her boundless enthusiasm for nutrition today.) Food was the focus of her household. She remembers sitting down to a Thanksgiving dinner that

mind body spirit

would have fed the Mayflower, feeling completely stuffed, only to clear the table, and with paper and pencil in hand, begin planning the family Christmas menu.

When Joan graduated from high school she went to work for a baking company. She stopped cheerleading, and within a year or so she began to slowly expand and take on the look of "the Pillsbury Doughgirl," in her words. So, like so many other people in that situation, she went on a diet and took off the weight. In the process, she got hooked on nutrition.

Joan worked on a degree in nutrition and then enrolled in Boston University, where she got a master's degree in clinical nutrition. She became a registered dietitian and is now a professor at Boston University's nutrition program. She also counsels individuals about changing their eating habits at her private practice. "I want people to know that good nutrition and healthy eating can be a fun and easy component of your day, not stressful," Joan says. "What I like to do is help people to eat right without it feeling like a part-time job."

Joan is a regular guest on TV and radio programs. She is also a member of the ABC News Medical Expert Network, a group of resource and on-camera experts for the ABC News Network, including Good Morning America, World News Tonight, 20/20, Nightline and ABC.com (the online service).

No More Excuses workshops

MY MISSION IS TO MAKE CHANGES IN PEOPLE'S LIVES. When I became serious about losing weight, I learned that losing weight is not just about diet and exercise. What I learned is that in order to make a lifestyle change, I had to alter the way I would think, feel, and live my life. Once you make the decision to change your life, you are no longer the old person with the same old challenges and problems, but a new person with a new attitude and a new way of doing things. I also realized I needed a whole new support group. The Connectors represent one step I took to provide the support I needed. They have kept me focused. And when I am in any given city, anywhere, I make a point of meeting with Connectors to make that important and valuable direct, personal contact.

There is something very nurturing and supporting when you get together with a group of people of like mind, spirit, and purpose. I would love to see you at one of my workshops and welcome you into the extended family that makes up the Connector spirit.

The Workshop
Workshops vary in length from 1-day, to 3 to 6 hour events, depending on the needs and desires of your group. I can customize my workshops to emphasize certain aspects for special groups or organizations. The emphasis is on motivation, inspiration and encouragement with a discussion of such topics as getting started, workout programs, food choices, staying focused and committed for life, and much more.

For date and times of workshops in your area, or for further information, watch the **www.connectingconnectors.com** web site or call: **1-800/460-8604**

mind body spirit

INDEX

mind 🏃 body 🏃 spirit 🏃

mind body spirit

mind body spirit

"Women are just beginning to shine their light and will continue to do so in the new millennium," asserts Valerie Bates, co-author (with Mark Yarnell and John Radford, Ph.D.) of Self-Wealth: Creating Prosperity, Serenity, and Balance in Your Life (Paper Chase Press). In her book, Bates provides the tools that women can use to break free and achieve their personal goals-without paying the price of their own inner peace and balance. Bates proposes that you can have happiness in all areas of your life, and tells you how to develop and use the latest self-mastery and peak-performance skills to do just that. She and her co-authors reveal:

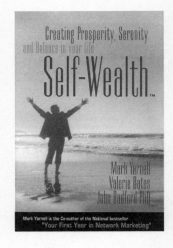

- *The advantages of setting goals larger than yourself*
- *The science of self-efficacy*
- *The nine principles of self-wealth*

In the past, authors such as Napoleon Hill, Norman Vincent Peale, and Tony Robbins have offered basic information about personal achievement. Bates and her coauthors build on those insights to reveal new, more advanced, scientifically proven ways to achieve both success and balance in your life. According to Bates, Self-Wealth could very well be the new Think and Grow Rich of the 21st Century!

$21.95, hardcover, 224 pages. Available in bookstores, from Amazon.com, or directly from Paper Chase Press at 800-460-8604.

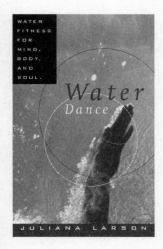

Water Fitness is changing lives! Juliana Larson explains why and shows people how to make it work for them.

- *Why choose water fitness over other traditional exercise programs?*
- *Can water fitness be used with cross training?*
- *What are the emotional and spiritual benefits of water?*
- *What is womentoring?*

Juliana Larson lovingly uses her expertise and inspiring stories of women to demonstrate water's positive effects on mind, body, and soul, provoking positive life changes. Water Dance opens the door for all, young and old, to entirely new ways of nurturing themselves and one another, improving their lives in the process.

$14.95, paperback, 224 pages. Available in bookstores, from Amazon.com, or directly from Paper Chase Press at 800-460-8604.